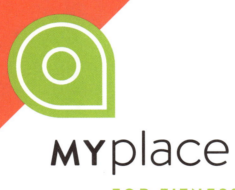

MYplace

FOR FITNESS

Published by First Place for Health
Galveston, Texas, USA
www.firstplaceforhealth.com
Printed in the USA
© 2018 First Place for Health

Cover design by Faceout Studio, Tim Green
Interior text design by Faceout Studio, Amanda Kreutzer

ISBN 978-1-942425-25-0

Caution: The information contained in this book is intended to be solely for
informational and educational purposes. It is assumed that the First Place for Health
participant will consult a medical or health professional before beginning this or any other
weight-loss or physical fitness program.

It is illegal to copy any part of this document without permission of First Place for Health.

To order copies of this book and other First Place for Health products in bulk quantities,
please contact us at 800.727.5223 or on our website: www.firstplaceforhealth.com

All Scripture quotations, unless otherwise indicated, are taken from the Holy Bible, New
International Version®, NIV®. Copyright © 1973, 1978, 1984, by Biblica, IncTM. Used by
permission of Zondervan Publishing House. All rights reserved worldwide.

Scripture quotations marked MSG are taken from THE MESSAGE, copyright © 1993, 1994, 1995,
1996, 2000, 2001, 2002 by Eugene H. Peterson. Used by permission of NavPress. All rights
reserved. Represented by Tyndale House Publishers, Inc.

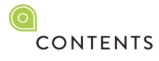

CONTENTS

Welcome to *My Place for Fitness* 6
About the Author 8
Why Christians Should Be Physically Fit 10
Your Body, Your Mindset 12
Discovering Your Why 19
A Quick Assessment 28
Know Your Fitness Numbers 38
How to Take Before-and-After Photos 47
FITT to Be Fit 48
The Activity Pyramid 54
A SMART Way to Begin 62
The Fitness Top 12 64
A Healthy Body Image 69
Where Do I Begin? Understanding the Types of Cardiovascular Training . . . 73
Strength Training 101 77
Flexibility and Balance Training 84
5 Fitness Myths We Need to Let Go Of 90
Activity Tracker—Do I Really Need One? 92
No Time to Work Out? Try HIIT 94
Water: The Everyday Guzzle 106
Get Out There and Walk! 110
Fit Your Feet—10 Tips for Choosing the Right Athletic Shoe for You 119
Born to Run? 123
Lacing Your Shoes for Comfort 124
Bicycling Your Way to Health and Fitness 130

5 Reasons You Aren't Losing Weight: Plateaus, Stalls and All-Out Standstills—How to Break Through	136
Making a Splash	138
Taking It Outside!	142
How to Look Chic During Your Workout	145
Staying Active on the Job	147
The Importance of Rest	150
Creating a Family Fitness Plan	152
Better Together—Working Out as a Couple	154
Choosing Home Gym Equipment	157
Gym-Bag Essentials	159
Staying Active While Traveling	161
Why and How to Choose the Best Personal Trainer for You	164
Turn off the Tube	172
Cause for Celebration	173
Glossary of Terms	174
Bibliography	180
Endnotes	182

MYplace O FOR FITNESS

WELCOME TO *MY PLACE FOR FITNESS*

I have to confess: I'm not the kind of fitness instructor who naturally pops out of bed in the morning, throws on my workout clothes, and can't wait to start working out. I'd much rather lie in bed and lazily get up, grab a cup of tea, spend some time in Scripture, and slowly welcome in the day.

I didn't grow up in a family that was passionate about exercise. My father suffered from a congenital heart defect and my mom was a schoolteacher who was on her feet all day and had four children at home to keep up with. The last thing either of them thought about was exercise.

But I do get up in the morning, throw on my workout clothes, and drive to the gym at 6:30 am to teach fitness classes. Why? Because I choose to. I choose to because I learned along my journey of life the value of exercise. I choose to because I watched my mom leave this earth from diseases that were preventable and treatable with physical activity. I choose to because I believe it honors God.

Do you not know that your bodies are temples of the Holy Spirit, who is in you, whom you have received from God? You are not your own; you were bought at a price. Therefore, honor God with your bodies

—1 Corinthians 6:19-20, NIV

Our goal through *My Place for Fitness* is to inspire you to choose fitness. We pray it will help you develop your own personal fitness strategies so that you can begin making changes starting today. We want to give you an understanding of fitness that will motivate you to choose a new level of health and wellness.

We also want this book to be a place where you can be real with yourself about your struggles and successes. We want you to write, pray, examine, and track your journey. Because although we can give you the tools, this is the place where the rubber meets the road. You are either going to do it or not. Some of you are excited about this journey and others of you might be dreading it. For those dreading it, First Place for Health believes that even small beginnings can yield tremendous results. We aren't going to ask you to go out and run a marathon tomorrow. We want you to start right where you are.

WELCOME

Someone once said, "A fit body is always under construction." It's not something you can achieve and then forget about. The old adage "use it or lose it" is true. We want to provide you with the tools and knowledge you need to attain and maintain an active lifestyle throughout your life. You are never too old, too heavy, too (fill in the blank) to start.

A few things you'll learn are:

o the benefits of physical activity

o the FITT formula

o how to determine your heart rate

o how to determine what exercise is right for you

o how to monitor your exercise intensity

o the importance of balance and flexibility

o how to choose a personal trainer

o and so much more

Zig Ziglar once said, "You don't have to be great to start, but you have to start to be great."

Today you've made a choice by opening this book. Congratulations! That's the first step toward change.

> *Therefore, I urge you, brothers and sisters, in view of God's mercy, to offer your bodies as a living sacrifice, holy and pleasing to God—this is your true and proper worship*
> —Romans 12:1

ABOUT THE AUTHORS

Vicki Heath is National Director of First Place for Health. Vicki is a certified fitness instructor for the American Council on Exercise, a certified life coach and Wellness Coordinator for her church in Edisto Beach, SC. Vicki is an author of the books Don't Quit Get Fit and Wellness Journey of a Lifetime. She has led a successful First Place for Health ministry in her church for twenty years. Vicki is passionate about Christ and has a desire to help others understand the value of caring for their bodies as temples of the Holy Spirit. Vicki is a pastor's wife and mother of four wonderful children and six grandchildren. She strives to bring others into the Kingdom through health and wellness.

Mary Ward has been teaching fitness classes for most of her adult life. She is a certified group fitness instructor through American Council on Exercise (ACE) as well as an ACE faculty member leading various Continuing Education classes for fitness professionals. She currently teaches Boot Camp, Power Strength, Cardio/ Strength, Gold and Dance Blast classes for Body & Soul Fitness. She is also certified with Refit Revolution. Mary is the Marketing Director with Body & Soul as well as leading the Northern Virginia Instructor Area.

When not teaching fitness classes, Mary is the CEO of Integrity Enterprise Solutions (IES), providing professional services to the federal government. She is also honored to sit on the Board of Directors for First Place 4 Health.

Mary's philosophy is "Don't think about why you can't, think about how you can."

WELCOME

WHY CHRISTIANS SHOULD BE PHYSICALLY FIT

Keep your eyes on *Jesus*, who both began and finished this race we're in. Study how he did it. Because he never lost sight of where he was headed—that exhilarating finish in and with God—he could put up with anything along the way: cross, shame, whatever. *And now he's there, in the place of honor, right alongside God. When you find yourselves flagging in your faith, go over that story again, item by item, that long litany of hostility he plowed through. That will shoot adrenaline into your souls!* —Hebrews 12:2-3, MSG.

Dr. Richard Couey, a former member of the President's Commission on Physical Fitness and Sports, an exercise physiology consultant for the U.S. Olympic Team, and a professor emeritus of health sciences at Baylor University in Waco, Texas, answers this question this way, "Christians should be physically fit this way: because Jesus was fit."

During His ministry on earth, Scripture says that Jesus walked from Sidon to Tyre between sunup and sundown, which equates to 52 miles. To do this He would have had to keep a 14-minute-mile pace. In fact, based on scriptural accounts, the total miles Jesus would have walked during His ministry would have been 3,125 miles in a 3-year period. You have to be fit to accomplish that.

Luke 2:52 says that Jesus grew in wisdom and stature, and in favor with God and man.

Dr. Couey gives us several reasons why we should, like Jesus, be fit. First, our Savior was fit. Jesus grew in all areas, in a balanced manner:

o Mentally—wisdom

o Physically—stature

o Spiritually—God

o Socially—man

If our desire is to be like Christ, then we must do the same. Ephesians 5:1-2 says, "Therefore, be imitators of God, as beloved children; and walk in love, just as Christ

MY JOURNEY

also loved you and gave Himself up for us, an offering and a sacrifice to God as a fragrant aroma." Neglecting one area will affect another.

Second, our bodies are God's creation.

- Genesis 1:1: "In the beginning God created the heavens and the earth."

- Genesis 1:9: "And God saw that it was good."

- Genesis 1:27: "So God created mankind in his own image, in the image of God he created them; male and female he created them."

- Genesis 1:31: "And God saw all that he had made, and it was very good."

Our bodies contain about 100 trillion cells that have 100,000 chemical reactions a second. Each cell has a nucleus that contains chromosomes that contain genes, and within each gene is our DNA. If we multiplied the length of each gene (17") by the number of genes on each chromosome (40,000) by the number of chromosomes (46) by 100 trillion, our DNA would reach to the sun and back more than 200 times.

Dr. Couey says, "God doesn't make no junk, but we're putting junk into God's creation."

And finally, scriptural principles: First Corinthians 6:19-20 says, "Do you not know that your bodies are temples of the Holy Spirit, who is in you, whom you have received from God? You are not your own; you were bought at a price. Therefore, honor God with your bodies."

- Ownership—Whose body is it? God's body; you received it from God.

- Occupancy—Who is in your body? That ought to be enough. You are carrying around God in your body, the Holy Spirit who is in you.

- Obedience—Show honor and glory to God with your body.

You can do this! "I can do all things through Him who strengthens me"
—Philippians 4:13

MYplace O FOR FITNESS

YOUR BODY, YOUR MINDSET

"I am fearfully and wonderfully made, your works are wonderful, I know that full well"

—Psalm 139:14

The act of getting strong doesn't start in the gym. It starts in your head.

A few years ago an exhibit came to town called BODIES. It was a display of real bodies (cadavers) that allowed each of us a glimpse into what the insides of our bodies looked like. I was so excited. I was going to get to see firsthand what the muscles I teach people to strengthen look like. I'm not sure what I expected to see when I walked in, as there was no skin on the bodies, but it didn't take long before I was mesmerized by how they had positioned each body into active movements so that it highlighted a specific set of muscles. Triceps, biceps, abdominals, quadriceps, gluteals, hamstrings and, my favorite, lattisimus dorsi on beautiful display for all to see. I was in muscle heaven.

It's hard to look at these bodies with all their detail and not believe that there is a God who created us in the most intricate way.

Our bodies are made of 206 bones, 608 muscles, 800 nerves, 100,000 miles of blood vessels, and 80-100 trillion cells. We have ligaments, muscles, joints and sinews that help us bend and move. Our bodies were made to be active.

I walked away from the exhibit even more fully convinced of how completely, fearfully and wonderfully we are made.

For much of man's history, being physically active was a part of life. We plowed fields, picked the harvest, rode horses or walked. We kneaded bread, hand washed clothes, and built our own houses. Our lives depended on physical work to sustain us. We didn't have the modern conveniences we have today, such as washing machines, microwaves, cars, planes, or computers. And unfortunately, as we've traded time for convenience, we've become much less active and our health has become the victim.

According to the State of Obesity Report 2016, too many of us are living sedentary lives. And it's literally killing us.

Consider these statistics:

- Physical inactivity is responsible for 1 in 10 deaths.

- 80% of adults don't meet the recommended guidelines for physical activity.

- 60% are not sufficiently active to achieve health benefits, up 15% from last year.

- Sedentary adults pay $1,500 more per year in healthcare costs than do active adults.

- There has been an 83% increase since 1950 in sedentary jobs.

My husband works at a desk. We were discussing the "number of steps per day" needed to maintain a reasonable level of fitness. He believed that because he was walking in and out of the office building, walking and talking to people throughout the day, attending meetings, and climbing stairs occasionally, he was averaging the guidelines of 10,000 steps per day.

I challenged him to wear a pedometer over the course of a week and track his daily steps. At the end of the week the results were in. He was walking around 2,500 steps a day.

Wow, sometimes we need an awakening. Are we really doing what we think we are and is it accomplishing what we hope?

The basic definition of physical activity is movement. This can include shopping, gardening, cleaning the house, traveling, climbing the stairs, even working can be physical activity if you do most of it standing on your feet or getting out of your chair often. It also includes exercise.

Exercise is a subset of physical activity. It is deliberate. It's something you plan to do. Exercise is an intentional decision.

The other day a friend said to me, "Whenever I see you, I feel convicted." I asked why. He said, "Because you're a fitness instructor, and just seeing you reminds me that I'm not exercising."

New studies are being done every day and not one of them has discovered that sitting down is beneficial to our health. In fact, they confirm the exact opposite: physical activity yields a long list of health benefits.

MYplace O FOR FITNESS

Let's take a look at just a few of the *physical* rewards.

(Circle those that are most important to you.)

Weight loss and weight control	Increased muscle strength and muscle mass
Increased metabolism	Increased energy
Increased "good" cholesterol	Improved flexibility and movement
Lower risk of a heart attack and stroke	Lower risk of some types of cancer (breast, colon, uterine-lining, and prostate)
Smokers quit with higher success rates	Reduced risk of type 2 diabetes and metabolic syndrome
Decreased risk of osteoporosis	Improved immune system

And these are just a few of the benefits! As scientists continue to study the body, more and more benefits are discovered daily.

So then, what are the governmental guidelines?

For major health benefits, the government recommends you do the following:

- 30 aerobic minutes of moderate intensity 5 times per week, or 25 minutes of vigorous intensity 3 times per week. These minutes can be broken up into three 10-minute segments throughout the day with the same benefits.

- Strength-train at least two days a week with a day of recovery in between workouts.

For even more health benefits, simply double the aerobic guidelines. (Remember to check with your doctor before starting a new exercise program, especially if you haven't exercised in a while or have any health concerns or chronic health issues.)

A gray-haired old lady, a long-time member of her community and church, shook hands with the minister after the service one Sunday morning. "That was a

MY JOURNEY

Here's even more good news—the long list of *mental health* benefits.

(Circle the ones that would add the most benefit to your life.)

Enhances the ability to handle daily stress and tension	Improves quality of sleep
Increases levels of serotonin and dopamine in the brain, which is linked with improved mood	Is associated with higher self-esteem and better body image
Increases endorphins, or the "feel good" chemicals in the body, which again improves mood and energy	Increases enthusiasm for life
Decreases symptoms of PMS and depression in women	Leads to a higher-quality sex life
Reduces anxiety and panic attacks	Improves better thinking, learning, and judgment in middle age and beyond

wonderful sermon," she told him, "just wonderful. Everything you said applies to someone I know."

You get the point. Most of us have heard about the benefits of exercise, and we know it's good for us, but we just don't do it. It's great for other people, but we make excuses and find reasons not to exercise ourselves.

On a scale of 1 to 10, how active are you?

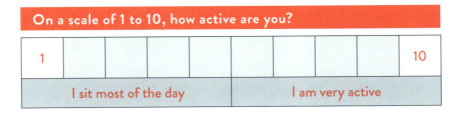

Any activity is better than none. If you are inactive, slowly increase your activity level. Even 60 minutes of moderate-intensity aerobic activity per week provides health benefits. Remember, your goal is long-term success. If you reach too far, too soon, you are more likely to injure yourself or drop out.

15

MYplace ○ FOR FITNESS

But why can some easily make a decision and move forward with excitement and some never seem to be able to get started?

One answer is mindset.

When it comes to mindsets, people usually fall into one of two categories: (1) a fixed mindset—what you were born with is what you have for life; it really can't be improved upon; or (2) a growth mindset—what you were born with can grow, develop, and be improved upon.

In her book *The Wellness Journey of a Lifetime*, *First Place for Health* National Director and author Vicki Heath says that we often take a backward approach to change. We change our behavior in hopes that it will change our thinking and eventually our mindset. But she challenges us to reverse the order. Change the mindset, which will change our thinking, which will change our behavior.

What is your mindset? Write it down here. Does it need to change?

_____

_____

_____

_____

_____

In First Place for Health, we believe that the change in mindset comes when we put God first in our lives. God's truth transforms, and it transforms us from the inside out.

In *The Message*, Eugene Peterson writes Romans 12:2 this way:

So here's what I want you to do, God helping you: Take your everyday, ordinary life—your sleeping, eating, going-to-work, and walking-around life—and place it before God as an offering. Embracing what God does for you is the best thing you can do for him . . . Instead, fix your attention on God. You'll be changed from the inside out. Readily recognize what he wants from you, and quickly respond to it. Unlike the culture around you, always dragging you down to its level of immaturity, God brings the best out of you, develops well-formed maturity in you.

Don't you love the promise of God's Word? When we fix our attention on God, we'll be changed from the inside out, transformed. God brings the best out of us—inside out. I love that our God is in the business of transforming us.

And while we read this verse considering our spiritual side, the principle applies to our physical bodies as well. Transformation begins inside before you see the results outside. I have to burn the fat inside of me before I fit into a smaller size pair of jeans. I have to strengthen the muscles inside of me in order to see a change in the things I can do physically.

Scripture says in Hebrews 12:11-12 that "no discipline seems pleasant at the time, but painful. Later on, however, it produces a harvest of righteousness and peace for those who have been trained by it. Therefore, strengthen your feeble arms and weak knees." It's a process. If you do the work, you will reap the reward.

If mindset is the first thing we need to change, do you believe you can develop a physically active lifestyle? Do you believe Scripture when it tells you that God will give you everything you need, even in the area of fitness?

Journal a few thoughts about what you saw modeled in your home growing up when you think of physical activity or exercise. Does it bring back fond childhood memories? Were you physically active at one time in your life and now find yourself sedentary? What caused the change?

_____

_____

_____

_____

_____

MYplace O FOR FITNESS

How do you feel when you hear the words "physical activity" and "exercise"?

As you look back over your thoughts, what stands out?

If you have never done it before, you are invited right now to choose to put God first in this area of your life and ask Him to transform your mindset, thinking and behavior. Ask Him what needs to change and make it your prayer.

DISCOVERING YOUR WHY

No time, no fun and bo-o-o-ring! These are three common reasons people give for not making physical activity a lifetime habit.

We all do it. We find excuses to get out of something we don't really want to do. I'm guilty of it myself. As a fitness instructor, I have given in to the occasional excuse to get out of exercise. I'm embarrassed to admit that my lamest excuse is that it will ruin my hair.

What's your favorite e.1xcuse? Is it one of the top 10 excuses people give as a reason to not work out?

1. I don't have time to exercise.
2. I don't live near a gym.
3. I don't know how to exercise.
4. I don't have the energy to exercise.
5. I don't have a buddy to work out with.
6. I don't like to sweat.
7. It's boring.
8. It's too hot/cold.
9. I'm too old.
10. It's no fun.

OK, so which ones are you guilty of? Can you list more? Some people call them reasons, but there is a big difference between reasons and excuses. Reasons are grounded in facts, whereas excuses are grounded in blame and untruths. Untruths are lies.

In her book *Don't Quit, Get Fit*, author Vicki Heath lists over 37 actual excuses that she has heard over the years as a fitness instructor and health and wellness coach. (I encourage you to make this book a part of your health and wellness library.) I won't list all 37 excuses, but my favorite is "my fat wiggles when I run."

If you, like me, have ever been guilty of this, then let's switch our mindset from excuses to reasons and find our why. Everyone has one; you just need to discover it.

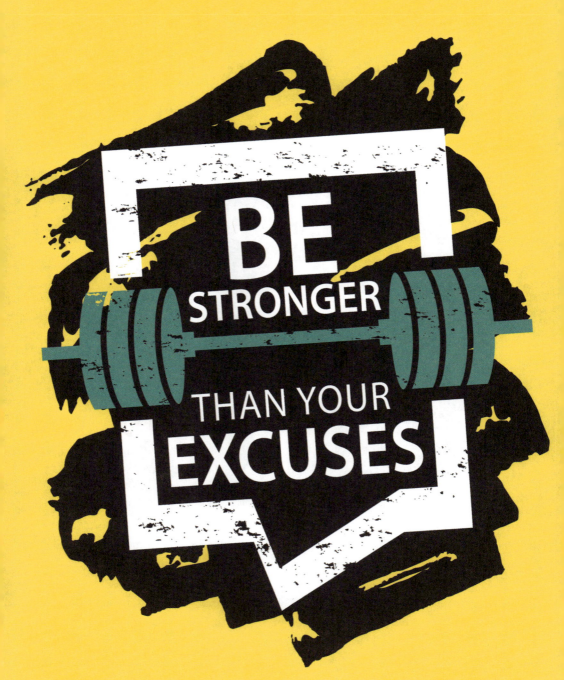

MY JOURNEY

The why will become your reason to succeed—your motivation, your drive. Without it you'll find yourself abandoning your program before accomplishing your goals.

Ask yourself these questions and see which rings true for you:

○ Do I want to be healthier?

○ Do I want to lose weight?

○ Do I want to become stronger?

○ Do I want to be fit enough to meet a goal?

Let's add two words to the questions above and see if they begin to change the answer: "But *why* do I want to . . . ?"

Dig down for your true motivation. Continue to ask yourself these questions over and over until you find your real reason. Short-term goals, such as an island vacation, a wedding, or a reunion, aren't going to give you the long-term results you really hope for. Your why often has an emotional component: you were teased as a kid, a loved one had a health issue, or possibly you had hard past experiences, such as abuse.

Are you worried that you might develop a health problem? Have you already developed one and you are afraid of what might happen to you? Are you tired of being the brunt of jokes and you want to rise above the ridicule? The discovery of your why might be the single most important piece to getting out of bed, putting on your fitness clothes, and working out. It can become the one thing that pushes you harder, challenges you the most, and takes you far past where you thought you could go. Let's see this play out.

Meet Christi. Christi is a married 42-year-old with three children. She is a working mom, involved with her kids' activities, and active in her church. Christi went to the doctor and was told that, in addition to changing her diet, she needed to exercise—that by doing so, she could reduce some of the risk factors the doctor was seeing in her test results. Her weight was higher than it had ever been and she was miserable. What Christi really wanted was the doctor to give her a quick fix and not tell her she needed to add more into her already busy schedule. Christi ignored her doctor's advice until a family reunion was coming up. Christi knew that she would be seeing people she hadn't seen in years and the thought of them seeing her at this weight had her feeling even more miserable and stressed. Christi thought back to her doctor's advice and started a fad diet and joined a gym. She lost 15 pounds and felt great for the reunion. She wanted to keep up with this new lifestyle.

Then her son broke his arm while playing football. Doctor visits and helping her son manage everyday tasks took her away from her new schedule. Before she knew it, she had gained 5 pounds, then 10. Soon Christi had put on 20 pounds. The holidays were coming up and family would be visiting. She rushed to buy gifts, plan meals, clean the house, and work. Christi found herself busy with life again and neglected herself.

Again, she thought back to her doctor. She determined to lose the now 20 pounds she gained. She started back at the gym and found a new diet. She lost 10 pounds and was happy enough. But another crisis hit and she stopped working out, ditched her new diet, and gained back the 10, plus more. Christi found herself not feeling well and went back to the doctor. He told her that her blood pressure was on the rise, her cholesterol was high, and she was now pre-diabetic. Christi was devastated.

Does any of Christi's story resonate with you? I've heard this story countless times. Sometimes we really desire change and even adjust our lifestyle to accomplish our goal. But then life takes an unexpected turn and our lifestyle change seems to go out the window.

Let's walk through Christi's story and see if we can move her beyond a short-term goal to a long-term lifestyle change by discovering her why.

We know this about Christi:

o   She wanted to lose weight.

o   Her weight was impacting her health.

o   She wasn't happy.

In discovering her why, the first question Christi needs to ask herself is this: "Why do I want to lose weight?" not "Do I want to lose weight?" The first question requires a real answer, while the second question can be answered with a yes or

MY JOURNEY

no. Let's say she answers, "I want to lose weight because I have a reunion coming up, I want to look good, and I'm stressed." She needs to follow this up with another question: "Why does the thought of others seeing me in my current state make me feel stressed and miserable?" The answer to this question can lead her to her why. In Christi's case, it revealed that others will see her perceived failure. Christi had been teased as a child, and an unkind remark from a teacher in front of her class had hurt her and left her embarrassed.

Christi finally realized that all change must come from within. She is now in the process of healing some old wounds and discovering her real goals—what she wants from life and why. This is helping Christi create lifelong change. She had never made herself a priority because she felt it would add stress to her life, but now she sees that neglecting herself has actually added stress. By implementing changes and planning for obstacles, Christi will accomplish all of her goals: she'll reduce her risk of disease, she'll be able to participate in any activity, she'll look better, and she will feel better about herself.

What could have been different for Christi had she learned what her why was earlier? What might she have avoided?

MYplace O FOR FITNESS

Josie is a 38-year-old who found herself over 300 pounds. Her 7-year-old son asked her one day, "Mom, why are you fat?" You can imagine Josie's reaction. It was time to get honest with herself. So Josie asked herself some questions to find her why: "Why am I fat? What do I want? And why is it important to me?"

She quickly came to her bottom line: she had become lazy. She didn't want her son to think of her as fat. She wanted to be a fit and healthy mom. But it was hard and it took time, and driving through the fast-food restaurant was easier than cooking. Sitting in the car during her kids' sports practices, catching up on email or social media, was easier than getting out and walking. She had developed a lifestyle of convenience and comfort that led to her being overweight.

Once Josie understood this, she put a plan in action that included small, simple steps at first. Making different food choices, putting down the phone, and walking during those practices began a new lifestyle for Josie. Over time she was able to lose more than 150 pounds and keep it off.

I've told you about my mother's health issues being part of my why. Why do I want to stay active? Because I want to avoid health conditions related to being sedentary such as diabetes and heart disease. But I also had to come to terms with some unforgiveness in my life. My need for forgiveness was for myself though, not for someone else. I hadn't forgiven myself for sin in my past. While I had gone to the Lord about it and knew I had His forgiveness, I hadn't forgiven myself and that needed to be dealt with. When I asked myself the questions of why, I came to the answer "because I don't deserve it." What a lie. But until I addressed it, I was stuck.

God doesn't ever want us to be burdened with shame and guilt. He wants us to walk in the true freedom that is found in Him. There are many scriptures that He could have used in my life, but during that time it was Psalm 32:1-5.

Take some time to discover your why. Ask yourself, "Why do I want to lose weight? Why do I want to be healthier? Am I simply living a lazy lifestyle? Is there anything I need to deal with—maybe a past hurt or a past sin?" Whatever it might be, take it to the Lord. Sit and reflect and confess whatever you need to. Ask Him for the strength and wisdom to develop a plan. Ask Him for a buddy or a coach who will help you meet your goals and stay on track. He is so faithful to forgive you, meet your need, and get you walking in freedom.

MY JOURNEY

Because of the Lord's great love, we are not consumed, for his compassions never fail. They are new every morning; great is your faithfulness

—Lamentations 3:22-23

MYplace O FOR FITNESS

For great is your love, reaching to the heavens; your faithfulness reaches to the skies

—Psalm 57:10

But you, Lord, are a compassionate and gracious God, slow to anger, abounding in love and faithfulness

—Psalm 86:15

I write these things to you who believe in the name of the Son of God so that you many know that you have eternal life. This is the confidence we have in approaching God: that if we ask anything according to his will, he hears us. And if we know that he hears us—whatever we ask—we know that we have what we asked of him

—1 John 5:13-15

"Commitment is staying loyal to what you said you were going to do long after the mood you said it in has passed."

—Author unknown

MY JOURNEY

MYPLACE O FOR FITNESS

A QUICK ASSESSMENT

"A bear, however hard he tries, grows tubby without exercise."
—A. A. Milne, *Winnie the Pooh*

My mother passed away from congestive heart failure due to heart disease and type 2 diabetes. I remember at almost every appointment the doctors advocating physical activity and exercise as part of her overall wellness plan. Why? They knew the tremendous impact it would have on her body. They knew that it had the potential to change her life and prolong her years.

The Centers for Disease Control and Prevention (CDC) defines physical fitness as "the ability to carry out daily tasks with vigor and alertness, without undue fatigue, and with ample energy to enjoy leisure-time pursuits and respond to emergencies." Fitness then is determined by the state of your heart, lungs, muscles, bones, blood pressure, blood sugar, energy level, brain, and mood, because it is these very things that allow us to live with vitality and strength—or not.

Given this definition, assess where you think you are right now:

In general, would you say your health is:

EXCELLENT	VERY GOOD	GOOD	FAIR	POOR

_____

_____

_____

_____

In the past week, how many days have you done at least 30 minutes of physical activity enough to increase your breathing rate?

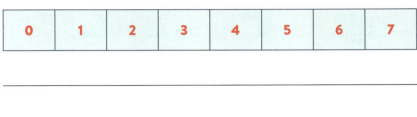

In the past week, how many days have you done strength training?

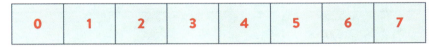

In the past week, how many days have you focused on stretching and flexibility?

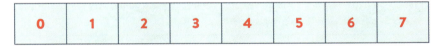

In the past week, how much physical pain have you experienced?

NONE	SOME	A LOT

MYplace O FOR FITNESS

On average, how much sleep do you get a night?

4 hrs	5 hrs	6 hrs	7 hrs	8 hrs	8+ hrs

Are you currently taking medications on an ongoing basis for cholesterol, high blood pressure, heart disease, or type 2 diabetes?

YES	NO

Have you experienced a major life change in the past year? (move, loss of job, death of a loved one, disability, etc.)

YES	NO

This assessment is personal to you. There is no pass or fail. It's a glance at where you currently are, whether you are just beginning or are a seasoned exerciser, and helps give you a starting point and, hopefully, motivation to move to the next goal.

For example, if you answered "fair" to the first question, what's your overall health goal and what steps can you take to get you to that goal?

If you answered "3" on the physical activity question, your next goal may be to get to "5."

What about your pain level? Does this keep you from exercising? Maybe your goal should be to incorporate flexibility and stretching into your routine.

What about sleep? Do you find yourself waking up tired? This alone can contribute to a lack of desire to exercise. It's important to evaluate sleep as an overall part of your fitness picture. A simple goal might be to increase the number of hours you sleep each night. Or you might talk to your doctor about a sleep study if taking steps to change your sleep habits hasn't worked.

What about stress? Being aware of your particular stresses will help guide you to make adjustments that will reap huge benefits. Psalm 46 starts by reminding us that "God is our refuge and strength, an ever-present help in trouble." It goes on to remind us to "be still and know that I am God." A goal might be to take time each day to sit still and pray.

Now let's do a more complete physical assessment. Four components play an important role in your overall health and fitness. A balanced fitness plan considers each of these areas:

1. Cardiovascular endurance (aerobic fitness)
2. Muscular strength and endurance
3. Flexibility
4. Body composition

Note to beginners: while these tests should not pose any special risk for most people, it's important to take a few precautions. If you have any underlying medical problems, such as heart disease or arthritis, talk to your doctor before taking any of these assessments. Don't push yourself to your maximum limit on any of these tests. The idea is to learn what you can do comfortably and then use the results to monitor your progress. As you prepare for the assessment, consider the following:

- Wear comfortable clothing and shoes appropriate for brisk walking.
- Avoid taking the tests on days when it's extremely hot, cold or windy.
- Have a friend or family member help you with the tests.

MYplace O FOR FITNESS

- Before beginning any tests, warm up for five minutes with light activity and stretching. Cool down when you have finished.

- If you experience any pain or discomfort during any part of the assessments, stop immediately and consult your physician.

How Aerobically Fit Are You?

There are a number of ways to assess your cardiovascular endurance and monitor your progress. One of the easiest and safest ways is to do a one-mile walk test.

What You Need

- A flat surface that allows you to measure off a one-mile distance, such as at a track at a local school, a walking path at a park, or at a shopping mall

- A stopwatch or watch with a seconds indicator to keep track of your time

What to Do

1. Practice taking your pulse several times before taking the assessment; then walk a mile as quickly as you can without straining.

2. At the end of the mile, record your time in minutes and seconds. Take your pulse for 15 seconds immediately upon stopping.

pulse = _____ Date _____

3. Multiply your pulse by 4 to get the number of heartbeats per minute.

pulse x 4 = _____ heartbeats/minute Date _____

I can walk one mile in _____ Date _____

Health-Related Fitness Standard: A good time is between 15 and 20 minutes (closer to 15 minutes if you're younger than 50). If you can walk the mile in less than 14 minutes, you're doing great.

MY JOURNEY

Recommendations: The only way to maintain your fitness level and get the health benefits you need is to be active on a regular basis. If you meet the aerobic fitness standard but not the activity standard, monitor your progress and repeat the test every 6 to 12 weeks. As your fitness improves you'll be able to cover the distance in less time.

How Fit Are Your Muscles?

Healthy muscles allow you to participate in a variety of activities with ease and enjoyment. Unfortunately, muscular fitness declines as we age. The only way to maintain healthy muscles is to exercise them on a regular basis. Take the following two tests to assess your muscular strength and endurance.

(1) CURL-UPS

This assessment tests the strength and endurance of the abdominal (stomach) muscles. Weak stomach muscles contribute to the lower-back pain that affects millions of adults.

What You Need

- A carpeted surface or an exercise mat

- A stopwatch or watch with a seconds indicator to keep track of your time

- We recommend a partner to hold your legs and count your curl-ups

What to Do

1. Lie on your back with your feet flat on the floor and knees bent at a 90-degree angle.

2. If you're a beginner, place your hands on your thighs and curl up slowly by lifting your shoulders off the ground. Continue to raise your body until your fingertips touch your knees. Don't lift up to a sitting position.

3. If you are already an exerciser, fold your arms at your chest and curl up slowly by lifting your shoulders off the ground. Continue to raise your body until your elbows touch your thighs.

4. Exhale during the upward movement and inhale on the way down. Don't hold your breath!

MYplace ○ FOR FITNESS

5. Do as many curl-ups as you comfortably can without straining. Stop at one minute.

I can do _____ curl-ups.   Date _____

Health-Related Fitness Standard: If you can do 15 to 20 curl-ups, you're doing well. If you can do 30 or more, you're doing great.

(2) PUSH-UPS

Doing push-ups is a good way to assess the strength and endurance of your upper body.

What You Need

○ A carpeted surface or an exercise mat

○ A stopwatch or watch with a seconds indicator to keep track of your time

○ We recommend a partner to count your push-ups and watch your form

What to Do

1. Lie face down with hands shoulders-width apart, palms face down and legs extended. Beginners should start in a kneeling position and can cross ankles. Hands should be directly under the shoulders as you begin the push-up.

2. Keeping your back and legs straight, push yourself up with your arms, shoulders and chest until your arms are straight, but elbow joint should not be locked.

3. Lower yourself back down until your chest touches the floor.

4. Exhale during the upward movement and inhale on the way down. Don't hold your breath!

5. Do as many push-ups as you comfortably can without straining. Stop at one minute.

I can do _____ push-ups.   Date _____

Health-Related Fitness Standard: If you can do 10 to 15 push-ups, you're doing well. If you can do 25 or more, you're doing great.

Recommendations: It's best to do at least one set of 8 to 10 repetitions that work each of the major muscle groups—shoulders, back, chest, arms and legs. You can do strength training using your own body weight, elastic exercise bands, hand and ankle weights, dumbbells, or machines.

How Flexible Are You?

Poor flexibility increases feelings of stiffness, limits mobility, and may increase the risk of certain injuries. Take the following test to assess your flexibility.

SIT AND REACH:

This assessment tests the flexibility of the backs of your legs (the hamstring muscles), hips and lower back.

What You Need

- A carpeted surface or an exercise mat

- A yardstick and strip of masking tape

- A partner to measure your stretch and watch your form

What to Do

1. Place the yardstick on the floor and put a long strip of masking tape across the yardstick at the 15-inch mark.

2. Sit on the floor with your legs extended, straddling the yardstick. Your feet should be 10 to 12 inches apart. Place your heels at the 15-inch mark with the 0 mark close to you.

3. With one hand on top of the other and fingertips even, slowly lean forward as far as you comfortably can along the yardstick. Exhale as you stretch forward and be sure not to bend your knees. Don't bounce or overstretch.

4. Perform the test three times and take your best measurement to the nearest inch.

Results _____   Date _____

MYplace **O** FOR FITNESS

Health-Related Fitness Standard: A good score is 12 to 18 inches. There's probably no health advantage to being able to stretch beyond these limits.

Recommendations: To increase or maintain your flexibility, perform several stretching activities at least three days each week; do them every day if you can. Never stretch to the point of pain, and avoid bouncing or jerking movements. Hold each stretch for 10 to 20 seconds. Avoid stretches that put pressure on your neck, lower back or knees.

Based on these assessments, my fitness goal is _____

MY JOURNEY

My overall goal is to _____

KNOW YOUR FITNESS NUMBERS

There are so many acronyms floating around the exercise world. You hear them all the time—BMI, BMR, WHR, MHR—but what do they all mean? Is one more important than the other?

You've started a new exercise program, but how do you know if you are working too hard or not hard enough? Will these acronyms be an important player in your new routine? They should!

Maximizing your efforts and working out safely are key. Determining your goals and being able to assess your own improvement puts you in the driver's seat. Knowing your body's limits as you exercise will give you the upper hand in creating an effective exercise plan and may be just what will get you through when you hit a plateau. Remember, its your personal journey.

There was a time when I didn't know what my target heart rate was. You know the common phrase "working up a sweat"? I thought sweat determined how hard I was working out. But did you know that sweating isn't really an indicator of this? Some can work out and never sweat (I'm so jealous), while others only have to think about working out and the sweat starts pouring (me). It's our own personal uniqueness. Once I figured out that I could take control of my fitness by arming myself with a little knowledge, everything changed.

Some common and less common terms you'll need as you start to begin to exercise, or look to improve your overall performance if you are already exercising, are the following:

RATE OF PERCEIVED EXERTION (RPE)—The Rate of Perceived Exertion scale is used to determine how you perceive the intensity you are feeling as you exercise. It is based on a number scale from 0-10. This is a great tool for beginners.

Zero would be as if you were sitting on the couch watching TV, while 10 would be very, very heavy activity. Beginners should strive to work at moderate activity level 4-6. For interval training, you want to shoot for 9 or 10 for the interval segment and use active rest, meaning move your feet or arms lightly, shooting for 2, during the rest segment. Using the RPE chart can really help you target each workout.

According to the American Council on Exercise, using the RPE method is more appropriate "for individuals taking certain medications that affect exercise heart rate, such as beta blockers for high blood pressure, and those with health conditions that affect heart rate, such as pregnancy."[1] It's also free, as opposed to purchasing a heart rate monitor, and you can quickly assess your workout level.

RATING OF PERCEIVED EXERTION

RPE		CATEGORY RATIO SCALE	
6		0	NOTHING
7	VERY, VERY LIGHT	0.5	VERY, VERY WEAK
8		1	VERY WEAK
9	VERY LIGHT	2	WEAK
10		3	MODERATE
11	FAIRLY LIGHT	4	SOMEWHAT STRONG
12		5	STRONG
13	SOMEWHAT HARD	6	
14		7	VERY STRONG
15	HARD	8	
16		9	
17	VERY HARD	10	VERY, VERY STRONG
18		*	MAXIMAL
19	VERY, VERY HARD		
20			

Source: Adapted, with premission, from American College of Sports Medicine (2000), *ACSM's Guidelines for Exercise Testing and Prescription* (7th ed.), Philadelphia; Lippincott Williams & Wilkin

RESTING HEART RATE (RHR)—Your resting heart rate is the number of times your heartbeats per minute at rest, literally. And not just any time of rest. You want to take it first thing in the morning, after a good night's sleep and before you get out of bed. Find your pulse at your wrist or the carotid artery on your neck. Using your index and middle fingers, press gently and count the number of beats you feel in 10 seconds. Multiply this number by 6 to find the number of beats per minute.

_____ x 6 = _____ RHR

According to the National Institutes of Health, the average resting heart rate for all adults (including seniors) should fall between 60 and 100 bpm.[2]

MYplace ○ FOR FITNESS

MAXIMUM HEART RATE (MHR)—Everyone has a maximum heart rate. When your heart reaches its limit, the muscles can't get all the oxygen they need, so your body has to slow down. Fortunately, it's not necessary to work at this maximum level to get the benefits of aerobic exercise. Most people don't know their true maximum heart rate (some fitness centers provide testing); however, you can calculate your predicted maximum heart rate. It's easy to compute. Simply take 220 and subtract your age. This is your maximum heart rate (MHR).

220 -_____ = _____ = MHR

It is recommended that you work within 55 and 85 percent of your MHR for 20 to 30 minutes to get the best results from exercise.

TARGET HEART RATE (THR)—Once you know your RHR and MHR, you can easily determine your target heart rate. While it's a bit more complicated, this number will help you calculate the intensity level you are working at or desire to work at. For this we'll be using the Karvonen Formula.

Let's use, as an example, a person who is 35 years old with a resting heart rate of 64. Starting with 220, simply subtract the age: 220 - 35 = 185. Then subtract the RHR of 64: 185 - 64 = 121. Multiply this number by intensity. Based on the recommended guidelines for daily exercise, start by multiplying 55%. Using our example, the answer for this person would be 66. Then, last calculation, add back in the RHR of 64 to equal 130. Therefore, 130 bpm is the target heart rate (THR).

Again, knowing this number will help you maximize your exercise efforts. This baseline number is the lowest you want your heart rate to work as you exercise. Continue to multiply by various percentages—65, 75, and 80—to give you the target heart rates for steady-state exercising, such as brisk walking, swimming, biking, hiking. In order to achieve the desired results using HIIT (high-intensity interval training) workouts, you'll want to know your 85, 90 and 95 percentages, because the active phases require higher intensities while the active rest periods require minimal effort. Use the chart below to calculate your own THR. You may want to enter them using a pencil. As you improve your fitness level, these numbers will adjust. Review them periodically and chart your new numbers.

MY JOURNEY

DETERMINING YOUR PERSONAL TARGET HEART RATE (THR)

220 minus _____ (age) = _____ (MHR) minus _____ (resting HR) = _____

MULTIPLY INTENSITY	+ RHR	= THR
55% =	+	=
65% =	+	=
75% =	+	=
80% =	+	=
85% =	+	=
90% =	+	=
95% =	+	=

YOUR PERSONAL TARGET HEART RATE CHART

WAIST CIRCUMFERENCE (WC)—Waist circumference is the measurement used as an indicator of health risk associated with excess fat around your waist. The more fat you have around your waist compared to your hips, the higher the risk for developing type 2 diabetes, high blood pressure, or heart disease. To measure, start at the top of your hip bone, then bring the tape measure all the way around, level with your belly button. Make sure it's not too tight and that it's straight. Don't hold your breath while measuring. Your waist should measure no more than 40 inches for men and 35 inches for women.

My waist circumference is _____ Date _____

WAIST TO HIP RATIO (WHR)—As with WC and BMI, the WHR is used as a measure of several things:

- Overall health

- Risk of developing serious health conditions

- Measurement of obesity

- Predictor of mortality

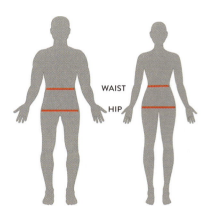

It's calculated as waist measurement divided by hip measurement (W ÷ H). To take the measurements, stand with your feet close together, arms at your side, and wear minimal clothing. Remain relaxed

and don't hold your breath. You'll want to take the measurements twice. If the results are within one centimeter of each other, use the average of the two. If the results are larger than one centimeter, retake the measurements.

To take the waist measurement, find the bottom of your rib cage. This should be the narrowest part of your waist. Using a measuring tape wrap the tape around this part of your waist. This is your waist measurement.

Enter your waist measurement: _____

Using the measuring tape, find the top of your iliac crest, or the widest part of your hip. Wrap the tape measure around this area of your hip. This is your hip measurement.

Enter your hip measurement: _____

OK, let's do the math.

Waist _____ divided by Hip _____ = _____ WHR

MEN	WOMEN	HEALTH RISK LEVEL
0.95 or less	0.80 or less	Low Risk
0.96 to 1.0	0.81 to 0.85	Elevated Risk
1.0 or higher	0.85 or higher	High Risk

Now that you have your personal WHR, let's talk about what it means for you and why it's important.

Body Mass Index (BMI) was once believed to be the gold standard in determining a person's obesity state. But in recent years, research has discovered that BMI alone is not enough. Knowing your WHR can tell you so much more about your overall health and risk of disease.

Higher levels of WHRs can be associated with the following:

- Stress

- Fertility problems

- Diabetes, or insulin sensitivities

- Cardiovascular disorders

- Hypertension

- High cholesterol

- Stroke

- Ovarian cancer in women

- Testicular and prostate cancers in men

- Cognitive abilities

The culprit is visceral fat. It's a deeper internal fat, and the more you have of it, the more damaging it is to your health.

Body shape does play a part in this. Apple shapes tend to be genetically prone to carrying more abdominal fat, while pear shapes carry weight in their thighs and buttocks. This makes apple shapes more at risk than pear shapes, but exercise plays a bigger role in reduction of visceral fat than was once thought.

However, a study conducted by researchers at Duke University Medical Center gives hope to those with apple shapes.[3] It found that people who were physically inactive had significant increases in visceral fat, and those who exercised had significant decreases in visceral fat over an eight-month period. This might seem like an obvious conclusion, but the study focused on exercise and diet. *Diet alone did not reduce visceral fat like exercise did.*

The study showed that "the control group that did not exercise saw a sizable and significant 8.6 percent increase in visceral fat in only six months," said Duke exercise physiologist Cris Slentz, lead author of the study. "We also found that a modest exercise program equivalent to a brisk thirty-minute walk, six times a week, can prevent accumulation of visceral fat, while even more exercise can actually *reverse* the amount of visceral fat."

What does this tell us? Exercise is more than just about losing weight. It is essential to your overall health and should be a key part of your overall health and wellness plan.

All this being said, let's take a look at Body Mass Index.

BODY MASS INDEX (BMI)—Body Mass Index is a ratio of weight in relation to your height. It's not a direct measurement of body fat and doesn't provide information about fat distribution. However, according to the National Institutes of Health, "BMI can be useful to measure a person's level of being overweight or obese. It is calculated from your height and weight and is an estimate of body fat and a good gauge of your risk for diseases that can occur with more body fat. The higher your BMI, the higher your risk for certain diseases such as heart disease, high blood pressure, type 2 diabetes, gallstones, breathing problems, and certain cancers.

- Although BMI can be used for most men and women, it does have some limits:

- It may overestimate body fat in athletes and others who have a muscular build.

- It may underestimate body fat in older persons and others who have lost muscle."[4]

To determine your BMI, use the following calculation, or simply search the internet for a BMI calculator. There are hundreds out there that will do it for you. Be sure to date your calculation so that you can chart your progress.

BMI = Weight in Pounds / (Height in inches^2) x 703

My weight_____ / my height^2 _____ x 703 = _____ date _____

BMI CATEGORIES:

- Underweight = <18.5

- Normal weight = 18.5–24.9

- Overweight = 25–29.9

- Obese = BMI of 30 or greater

BASAL METABOLIC RATE (BMR)—Each day your body expends energy just to function. It has to breathe, generate new cells, regulate your temperature, and digest food, to name just a few. Your BMR is the number of calories your body would burn if you stayed in bed all day. Knowing your BMR is important to know whether your goal is weight loss or improving your ongoing fitness routine. It gives you an idea of how much fuel you need to keep your body going all day long.

BMR decreases with loss of lean body mass (or increase of fat) and with age (2 percent per year after the age of 20) and the loss of lean body mass. A regular exercise routine of cardio and strength training can increase your BMR.[5] You can calculate your own BMR using the formula below or, as with the BMI, you can search for a BMR calculator on the internet.

MYplace O FOR FITNESS

For men: BMR = 10 x weight (kg) + 6.25 x height (cm) – 5 x age (years) + 5

For women:BMR = 10 x weight (kg) + 6.25 x height (cm) – 5 x age (years) – 161

My BMR is _____ date _____

RESTING METABOLIC RATE (RMR)—This is the body's rate of energy used early in the morning after an overnight fast and a full eight hours of sleep. This is different from BMR.

Here's the bottom line on your numbers: Exercise will positively affect your health by improving or lowering your RHR, increasing your BMR, decreasing your WC, WHR, BMI, and by gaining all of the benefits that come with it.

What's the measurement of success for your personal fitness journey? Just as tracking your food will help you achieve success, journaling the numbers we've just walked through can give you the data you need to stay encouraged, help you see the progress you're making, and ultimately reach your goals. You've worked hard to improve your fitness. Let yourself see it on paper.

TRACKING MY FITNESS NUMBERS		
DATES	RHR	MHR

MY JOURNEY

HOW TO TAKE
BEFORE-AND-AFTER PHOTOS

Photos are a great way to really visualize your progress. Take your before pictures the day you start your fitness program (or within the first week). Wear swimwear or tight-fitting workout wear. You want to see all the changes that have taken place in your body! But only show as much of your body as you are comfortable with. And remember to include your face in the picture too.

Stand in front of a plain wall with as little clutter behind you as possible. Take photos from many angles, including a front, side, and back view, and maybe add an angled twist. Ham it up—flex your arms in the air or place your hands on your hips! Or just let them hang by your side. Whatever pose you choose, make sure that you take the "after" photos in the same pose! And don't suck it in or push it out. You want to see the real transformation. Take progress pictures—wearing the same clothing—30, 60, and 90 days later.

Use a tripod or selfie stick if you want to take your own photos, or grab a friend or family member and make them part of your team! Once you've reached your goal, share your photos with us. We might use your story in one of our upcoming newsletters. Send your photo to myplaceforfitness@firstplace4health.com.

BMR	BMI	WC	WHR

MYplace O FOR FITNESS

FITT TO BE FIT

Have you ever put on your fitness clothes, determined to exercise, and then realized at the end of the day that you haven't changed your clothes and haven't worked out either? I have. I now live by the quote "Exercise in the morning before your brain figures out what you're doing." There are many benefits to getting your workout in first thing in the morning, but the bottom line is to plan. For me, I know that if I don't get it done first thing, then I probably won't get it in. That's where the FITT principle can come in.

The FITT principle is designed to be the foundation for building the optimal workout routine for you. It connects your experience and your goals to create a plan that is personalized and, honestly, makes it easier to accomplish.

First, ask yourself these questions:

Experience:

What's your current fitness level: novice or beginner, leisure exerciser, intermediate, or advanced?

_____

_____

_____

_____

_____

_____

_____

MY JOURNEY

Goals:

What do you want to achieve in the next 6 to 12 months in terms of your overall fitness? Is your goal to lose weight, increase your strength or muscle tone, build up overall endurance, or perhaps all of the above?

_____

_____

_____

_____

_____

_____

Knowing your starting point and what you want to achieve can help you apply the FITT principle.

- Frequency: "How often should I exercise?"

- Intensity: "How hard should I exercise?"

- Type: "What kind of exercise should I do?"

- Time: "How long should I exercise?"

The four questions or components are interdependent. For example, the type of exercise (cardio or strength) will affect your time and frequency; intensity will affect your time and frequency; frequency will determine your time, type and/ or intensity.

Let's break these down:

Frequency

"How often should I exercise?" The type of exercise is important to frequency. Cardio and flexibility can be done every day, while strength training should be done two or three times per week.

(Read "The Fitness Top 12.") Be realistic. The guidelines suggest 30 minutes, 5 days a week. What will your schedule allow and what are your goals? If you are new to exercise, a good goal to start with is two or three days a week. Then increase your number of days as you are able. With this scenario, include strength training with your cardio to maximize your effort.

If your goal is to lose weight and your fitness level allows, training five or six days a week might be the frequency to shoot for.

Build in a leisure day when your activity is spent on a favorite hobby, sport, or playing with kids/grandkids.

Intensity

"How hard should I train?" Consider your goals. We've already stated that the guidelines are 30 minutes, five days a week. Intensity can impact the time spent exercising. Therefore, the higher the intensity, the less time you might spend exercising. For example, the caloric burn of a 30-minute jog is equal to a 45-60 minute walk.

Interval training is a great example of this. It combines short bursts of intense exercise followed by rest periods, which provide fitness results that are similar to or better than steady-state exercise but in shorter periods of time. High-Intensity Interval Training (HIIT) is a type of interval training that is very popular today—and for good reason. The National Institutes of Health has more than a dozen studies[6] that focus on HIIT workouts for the obese population and have found them to be safe and effective for long-term weight loss for this population.

Your fitness level can also determine intensity, which is important to consider. If you are new to exercise, you want to know certain numbers (read "Know Your Fitness Numbers," page 36), such as target and maximum heart rates. You want to work safely. Knowing these will ensure that you are working hard enough but not overtraining. Intensity needs balance. It's the Goldilocks principle—finding the "just right" place that will give you your desired outcome.

Type

"What kind of exercise should I do?" Will you be doing cardio, strength training, flexibility, or a combination of all three? Frequency, intensity and time all factor into type. Each brings different requirements per week and is where you get to personalize your workouts for your level and ability.

Cardiovascular training focuses on increasing your heart rate to a desired level. Your heart is a muscle and, just like any other muscle, needs to be worked. Strength training builds and tones your muscles and bones through either muscle endurance or muscle strength. Flexibility lengthens and stretches your muscles to keep them limber, elastic and supple. Each is an important part of overall fitness.

Body-weight exercises, such as mountain climbing, combine cardio and strength training, getting more done in less time. Pilates or yoga combines strength training and flexibility. Combining different types of training is a great way to improve general fitness and maximize your time.

Time

"How long do I have to exercise?" Time will be based on the frequency, intensity and type of exercise. Consider your goals. Focusing on endurance will mean using longer steady-state workouts. If weight loss is your goal, the number of days will be as important as the number of minutes spent exercising.

Strength training requires a day of rest between workouts, which means you won't spend as much time strength training as you do on cardio. Muscles need to repair and rebuild on those in-between days. Strength training increases your metabolism, builds bone density, and keeps burning fat long after your workout is over. So don't skip this.

If you've done a day of combined training, take the next day to walk, swim, do Pilates, or stretch. Which brings us to flexibility. Flexibility is often overlooked but it's so important. It increases blood flow to the muscle, decreases your risk of overall injury, and increases your physical performance.[1] Take at least 10 minutes a day to stretch.

MYplace O FOR FITNESS

PUTTING IT ALL TOGETHER

Here's your chance to write your own personal FITT prescription. I like the word "prescription" because doctor's write prescriptions to make you feel better. Putting the FITT principle into practice should do exactly that—make you feel better. It should also be realistic and fun. Don't look at exercise as punishment for what you've done or not done to your body. Celebrate physical fitness/exercise for what you can do and what you can achieve today.

Cardiovascular Exercises

- Frequency: 3 to 5 days a week

- Intensity: 50 percent to 85 percent of target heart rate

- Type: Activities that use large muscle groups, can be maintained continuously, and are aerobic in nature

- Time: 20 to 60 minutes of continuous aerobic activity (minimum of 10-minute bouts accumulated throughout the day)

Strength-training Exercises

- Frequency: 2 to 3 days per week

- Intensity: A minimum of one set of 8 to 12 repetitions on each muscle group to the point of muscle fatigue

- Type: Separate exercises that use resistance to strengthen major muscle groups— arms, shoulders, core body, and legs—usually includes the use of free weights, circuit training, resistance bands, and/or body weight

- Time: 20 to 30 minutes for most individuals

Flexibility and Balance Exercises

- Frequency: Daily

- Intensity: Gentle stretching to the point of tension, never pain

MY JOURNEY

- Type: General stretches of all major muscle groups and tendons

- Time: 10 minutes, holding each stretch 10 to 30 seconds

Beginners: As you become more fit and active, increase the number of days you work out. Try for a daily combination of both lifestyle activity and programmed activity. Then increase the number of minutes you work out. If you are working out for 20 minutes, take it to 30. Before you know it, you'll be developing a daily habit of exercise.

Intermediate Exercisers: Discover the benefits of HIIT training or interval training. Pump up the weights. And don't neglect stretching and flexibility.

Remember what we've already said—small beginnings can yield huge benefits and too much too soon can result in injury. Your body needs time to repair and rebuild after any exercise session. The goal of exercise is to provide a greater load or stress on the body than it is used to in order to improve fitness. It's important to find a balance between that load and recovery. Always reevaluate your personal FITT prescription as you see improvement.

Note to self: Someday is not a day of the week.

R$_{\times}$

DATE _____

NAME _____

FREQUENCY _____

INTENSITY _____

TIME _____

TYPE _____

MYplace O FOR FITNESS

THE ACTIVITY PYRAMID

You may have heard the song "Better When I'm Dancing" by Meghan Trainor. I love the lyrics. They describe how effortless it is to dance, and that you can move with confidence. They say not to let the world hold you back, that you can be successful, and that exercise or movement doesn't have to be hard. It can be fun.

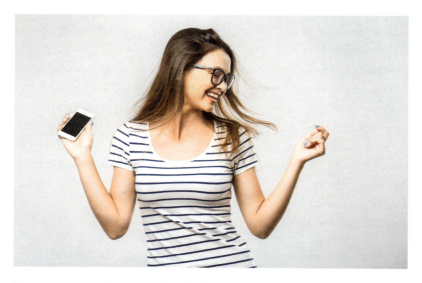

Since the song refers to dancing, let's take it as an example. Picture yourself at a wedding: the music starts to play, your foot begins to tap to the beat, your head starts to bob, and before you know it you're on the dance floor. You're moving without really even thinking about it.

So, what's happening inside your body when you dance? Your heart rate goes up, you're moving your joints, loading your muscles, engaging your core, burning calories, and having fun. And while dancing isn't a lifestyle activity for most people, the concept of incorporating more activities into your life that just get you moving should be.

There are a range of daily activities that offer the basis for good health. The activity pyramid, which is based on the recommendations of major health and fitness organizations, is a simple guide for visualizing how these can fit into your life. You don't have to dance unless you want to, but you can use this guide to choose what works best for you based on your goals, interests, abilities and lifestyle.

LEVEL OF THE PYRAMID

Lifestyle Activities

The base of the pyramid includes lifestyle activities that can easily fit into your daily routine. A lifestyle activity is one that increases your heart rate 4 to 7 times higher than your resting heart rate.

The good news is that lifestyle activities don't have to be done all at one time. Short periods of activity will result in health benefits as long as the total of the periods adds up to 30 minutes or more each day.

The following are some examples of lifestyle activities:

- climbing stairs instead of using the elevator

- doing housework

- working in your garden

- playing with the kids

- parking your car farther away

- walking the dog

- pushing a stroller

All of these are great ways to get started on a program of healthy everyday physical activity.

MYplace **O** FOR FITNESS

Look at the Activity Pyramid and list some improvements that you'll see in your own health by incorporating some of the lifestyle activities into your day. Which activities can you add easily?

MY JOURNEY

THE ACTIVITY PYRAMID

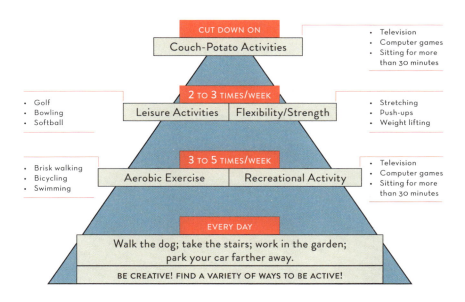

MYplace O FOR FITNESS

Aerobic Activities

The next level of the pyramid includes aerobic activities. This level follows the more traditional FITT prescription. Because aerobic activities are typically more vigorous, 20 minutes at least 3 days each week will provide benefits similar to those of daily lifestyle activities. As the variety, intensity and duration of activities increase, the health and fitness benefits increase. The more active you are, the more calories you burn.

The following are examples that fit into this category:

- group fitness classes

- swimming

- biking

- hiking

- running

- brisk walking

- dancing

- playing sports

- skiing and cross-country skiing

- treadmill/elliptical/stationary bike

Looking again at the Activity Pyramid. What aerobic activities can you add three days a week, and what are the improvements you might see in your own health by doing so?

Strength and Flexibility Activities

The third level of the pyramid emphasizes strength and flexibility exercises. Muscular strength and endurance are also important for overall health and quality of life. Strong muscles allow you to participate in a variety of daily activities with ease and enjoyment. Strength-building activities should be performed two to three days each week. Performing one set (10-12 repetitions) of several different exercises that use all the major muscle groups is all you need. You can use your own body weight, elastic bands or small hand-weights. Focus should be on major muscle groups, such as biceps, triceps, shoulders, abdominal, and back, and could incorporate squats, lunges, push-ups, and core exercises, to name just a few.

Flexibility is the ability to move the joints through a full range of motion. It reduces pain and stiffness, prevents injuries, and makes you feel better. Flexibility exercises should be performed every day, but a minimum of two to three days each week is acceptable. Focus on stretching all of the same major muscle groups that you are strength training.

MYplace **O** FOR FITNESS

Looking at the Activity Pyramid, how would you benefit in your own health by incorporating strength-training and flexibility activities into your life? List those benefits below.

_____

_____

_____

_____

_____

_____

At the top of the Activity Pyramid are things you should cut down on or do more sparingly, such as watching TV, playing computer or video games, or sitting for long periods of time doing activities like knitting or needlework. None of these things is bad, but when you find that these activities are causing you to be sedentary, just know that it will impact your health.

List some of the more sedentary activities you do that may have directly impacted your health in a negative way. What changes can you begin to make?

_____

_____

_____

_____

_____

MY JOURNEY

_____

_____

_____

_____

PUTTING IT ALL TOGETHER

Let's put this all together for you. In the diagram below, you're going to build your own activity pyramid. Transfer the things you listed above onto the pyramid. Lifestyle activities go at the base of the pyramid. The next level up is aerobic activities. Maybe you can only list one to start with. That's OK. Remember, we said to start slowly. Too much too soon can cause burnout or injury. Doing that one thing three days a week is a great beginning. Then level up and add strength-training and flexibility activities. This becomes your goal. Print it out and post it where you can see it daily as a reminder to keep moving.

THE ACTIVITY PYRAMID

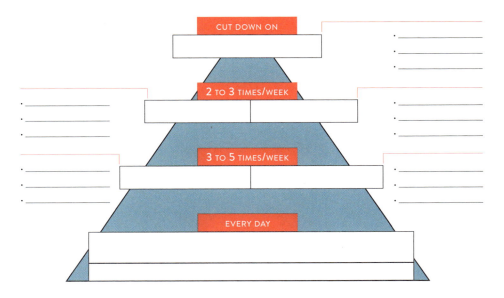

61

MYplace ○ FOR NUTRITION

A SMART WAY TO BEGIN

Are you ready for a change but aren't sure how to get started? Or maybe you've already set more goals than you care to admit but can't seem to reach them.

No matter how large or small your goal might be, creating change requires SMART planning. Whether you want to lose 5, 10, 25 or 50 pounds, walk a mile, run a marathon, or just be fit enough to play with your kids, following these guidelines may lead you to the success you've been desiring.

SPECIFIC—Your goal should be clear and easy to understand. A lot of people say they want to "get healthy" but this is too general. Instead, ask yourself, "Why do I want to get healthy?" A goal to exercise 30 minutes, 4 days a week is specific. It's a declaration of what you will do and for how long you'll do it.

MEASURABLE—A goal to "lose weight" is not enough. How will you track your progress and how you will know when you have reached your goal? Making your goal measurable means adding a number.

ACCOUNTABLE—One important piece of First Place for Health is the accountability. I've always been the strong-willed child who forged her own roads, but now I participate in an online group. I love it and wouldn't miss it. I have to admit that the first time I had to step on the scale and take a picture of my weight gave me pause. I didn't want to. But I've come to realize that it's just a number that is measuring my goal. It doesn't define me. I also send in my daily food trackers to our group leader and I'm beginning to realize its impact on the scale. When I track and send in my diary, it almost always results in weight loss. But the biggest part of being accountable that I have come to cherish is having a community that cheers me on. Having a team that accepts you where you are now, encourages you when your weight doesn't change, helps to keep you motivated when you want to give up, and prays for you? That can't be beat.

Maybe for you an online food journal is the beginning of accountability.

REALISTIC—Set goals that are realistic to where you are in your life right now. If weight loss is your goal, then what number is realistic? An overly aggressive goal might undermine your efforts. One hundred pounds might seem out of reach and overwhelming, but breaking it down to increments of 10 or 25 pounds might seem

MY JOURNEY

more manageable. If you are new to exercise, setting a goal to work out every day may not be realistic, but a goal of meeting the government standards for exercise might be.

TIMEFRAME—Having a time limit can prompt you to get started. Healthy weight loss is about 1-2 pounds per week, so set your timeline accordingly. For example, "I can lose 25 pounds in 6 months" or "I can lose 10 pounds in 2 months" are timelines that are achievable.

Now that you understand SMART goals, write down your goals and date it!

Today's Date	Target Date	Start Date

Specific	Know exactly what you want to accomplish. Use what, where, why, when, how questions.
Measurable	Establish how to measure success: actual members target dates, or specific events
Accountable	What tools will you use to remain accountable to your goal?
Realistic	Set goals you will be able to accomplish and consider any obstacles you may need to overcome.
Timeframe	Set a date you want to accomplish your goal by.

MY SHORT TERM GOAL:

MY LONG TERM GOAL:

DATE ACHIEVED:

THE FITNESS TOP 12

I remember saying to myself, "Where do I even begin?" when I started writing this book. This is when a few simple and practical steps provided the encouragement I needed to put a plan into action. I sought advice, outlined an approach, and started with Step 1.

You may be feeling the same way: "How will I ever be able to do this?" It's our hope that the Fitness Top 12 will help you to begin to formulate your own plan—starting with Step 1. As you work through the other steps, you'll begin to see a strategy develop that is uniquely yours.

Someone once said, "Success is not a big step in the future. It's a small step taken now." You've sought advice, you are outlining your approach, and you are starting at Step 1. You've got this!

Get Rid of Excuses

The word "excuse" comes from the Latin word *excusare*, which means to free from blame. Excuses can be dangerous to your success. They are lies designed to free you from feeling guilty about not doing what you know you should. Take a minute to list all the excuses that come to mind. As you look over your list, pray about each one, asking the Holy Spirit to guide you in determining which ones are lies and which ones you may need help in overcoming. The best defense is a good offense. Memorize 2 Corinthians 10:5. Make this your go-to Scripture when excuses try to creep in.

> *Success occurs when your dreams get bigger than your excuses.*

MY JOURNEY

Set Realistic Goals

What's more easily attainable: competing in an ironman race or walking one mile? Unrealistic and vaguely stated goals lead to exercise dropout. It's important to establish a training goal that is specific and appropriate for your fitness and skill level (do something a bit challenging but not overly difficult).

If you are a beginner exerciser, setting a goal to run a marathon might not be the best goal, maybe setting a goal to run/walk a 5K would be the better challenge. If you are already exercising and looking for that push, maybe participating in a 10K or taking a higher intensity fitness class would be a new challenge.

Keep in mind that we are all at different levels of fitness. Be honest about where you are now and realistic about where you want to get to. Look for a fitness coach or personal trainer who can help you determine your current fitness level and help you create a timeline for achieving the results you desire.

Make Physical Activity an Appointment

Have you ever heard the famous quip by Benjamin Franklin, "Those who fail to plan, plan to fail." Plan a daily time for your workout. Schedule it into your day and keep the appointment. This not only establishes the importance in you but also to the rest of the world that you are serious. "A good plan today is better than a perfect plan tomorrow"—some wise advice from the great General Patton. You get the point.

Do Something Every Day

Not having a full hour to exercise is no reason to skip your workout. Research shows that even three 10-minute exercise sessions a day can provide important health benefits.

Get up from your desk every 50 minutes and take a lap around the office or climb the stairs. Set your watch or alarm as your reminder, and before you know it, you'll have more than your 30 minutes of exercise in. And if every other day you make one of those 10-minute segments a strength-training workout, then you'll be in for a bonus. Need a meeting with a co-worker? Plan a walking meeting. Need to pray? Multitask and go for a prayer walk. Bad weather? Take it inside and walk the mall.

Find Something You Like to Do

Are you a people person? Find a group exercise class. A group will motivate you. And there are so many choices, from dance, to aqua, to HIIT, to boot camp, to martial arts, to spinning, to Pilates. Try out new classes until you find the ones you like best.

Are you someone who enjoys solitude, likes to be alone, or needs a detailed plan? You might benefit from time spent with a personal trainer who can guide you to a strategy that meets your specific needs.

Ask yourself what motivates you. Was there something you did as a kid that you really liked to do? This could be the start of a lifetime of enjoying physical activity.

Progress Wisely

Exercising too much and too hard is a common mistake that often results in injury. Rest after exercise. Gradually progress in time and intensity. This is one of the best ways to develop a routine that you will look forward to and not abandon.

Add Variety

Too many people find a routine or physical activity they like and then never vary from it. That might be OK for some, but doing the same workout every day can lead to boredom—which is one of the top four reasons people quit. There are so many choices out there. Mix it up and make it fun. Perhaps you can throw in a tennis game or a pick-up basketball game. There are all kinds of adult leagues that make physical fitness playtime—dodgeball anyone?

Find a Buddy

Studies show that those who exercise with a friend or group find more success and accountability. Asking a friend to join you might just be the motivation your friend needs to get moving. Pray and ask God to provide you with a buddy. Does someone immediately come to mind? Make a list of a few people you can workout with. One might like to dance while another might like to walk. Get them both on your team.

Invest in the Proper Shoes and Equipment

How long has it been since you bought a new pair of walking or workout shoes? If your answer is more than a year, you could be putting yourself at risk for injury. Investing in good shoes and other equipment will motivate you and keep you injury free.

Many stores have machines that will analyze your gait. Do you overpronate, underpronate, or have a neutral foot? These machines can answer these questions for you. And the best part about it is that you aren't obligated to purchase anything. Do yourself a favor and find out what shoe might be best for your feet.

Fitness trackers or heart rate monitors are great pieces of equipment to invest in. Heart rate monitors can help you meet your intensity goals by tracking the percentage of intensity you are working in. To track your daily progress, consider one of the many fitness activity trackers on the market today. Most will sync to your mobile technology, whether a phone or a tablet.

Expect to Become Weary

It's normal to come out of the gate running for about the first two weeks, and then *bam!* The newness wears off, the honeymoon is over, and your workout is nothing

MYplace O FOR FITNESS

but hard work. When you start your new program, expect this. We all become weary; but if you stay diligent and press on, you will reap wonderful benefits!

Learn from Past Failures and Successes

So many of us are unwilling to try for fear of failure. If you previously dropped out of an exercise program, it might not have been the right one for you. Try again, and evaluate your new routine as you progress. Michael Jordan said, "I've missed more than 9,000 shots in my career. I've lost almost 300 games. Twenty-six times I've been trusted to take the winning shot and missed. I've failed over and over and over again in my life. And that's why I succeed."

Celebrate Appropriately

Who doesn't love to be rewarded? We have awards for just about everything. So don't forget to reward yourself as you reach goals along the way. Do something special after you've walked your first mile, run your first race, attended your first water aerobics class. Reward yourself with a pair of new workout shoes, new work-out clothes, or a trip to your favorite getaway. Or how about a spa day?

Be creative: "I will reward myself with..."

_____

_____

_____

_____

_____

_____

_____

A HEALTHY BODY IMAGE

Let's start by reminding ourselves what God says about who we are:

Then God said, "Let us make mankind in our image, in our likeness...God saw all that he had made, and it was very good"
—Genesis 1:26,31

I praise you because I am fearfully and wonderfully made; your works are wonderful, I know that full well
—Psalm 139:14

For we are God's handiwork, created in Christ Jesus to do good works, which God prepared in advance for us to do
—Ephesians 2:10

Brothers and sisters, whatever is true, whatever is noble, whatever is right, whatever is pure, whatever is lovely, whatever is admirable—if anything is excellent or praiseworthy—think about such things
—Philippians 4:8

I have loved you with an everlasting love; I have drawn you with unfailing kindness
—Jeremiah 31:3

When we pick up any fashion magazine, flip on the TV, or notice the billboards lining the roadway, what do we see? Everywhere we turn, we're presented with unrealistic images of how we should look, what we should wear, and how we should live. Beautiful bodies are placed alongside ads for fattening foods, sending the message that you *can* have it all. It's crazy.

How do you measure up to what you see? How do these images and messages influence the way you feel about yourself? Do they influence your lifestyle habits and the goals you set for yourself? Do these messages and ideals line up with God's Word and what He says about you? Look back at the verses we just read.

We can't allow society's unrealistic expectations to influence the goals we set or the way we feel about ourselves. Trying to live up to these unrealistic demands will only lead to failure, guilt and disappointment. I believe God wants more for us than this. Theodore Roosevelt once said, "Comparison is the thief of joy." Isn't that so true? God's Word never asks us to compare our physical bodies to anyone. His Word tells us to "renew our minds and not conform to the pattern of this world" (Romans 12:1-2). His Word challenges us to "set your mind on the things above and not earthly things."

—(Colossians 3:2)

Achieving society's current ideal body image requires extremes of diet, exercise and cosmetic surgery; it's an image that often comes at the price of good health. Despite what we're led to believe, our society's version of the ideal body is outside the reach of the majority of men and women and is not a matter of self-discipline. There's absolutely no truth to the prevailing message that thinness equals health and happiness.

What the Numbers Show
- According to the North American Association for the Study of Obesity, 52 percent of men and 66 percent of women in America are unhappy with their weight. Studies show that 80 percent of women are dissatisfied with their appearance at one time or another.[1]

MY JOURNEY

- It is estimated that 40 to 50 percent of women are trying to lose weight at any given time. Many women on diets are already at or below a normal body weight.[2]

- In 2000, 79 percent of Americans reported that they were trying to lose weight through dieting. However, most were not incorporating recommended weight-loss strategies.[3]

- According to the U.S. Centers for Disease Control and Prevention, the average man is 5'9" tall and weighs 195 pounds; the average woman is 5'4" tall and weighs as much as the average man did in the 1960s—168.7 pounds. However, the average female fashion model is between 5'9" and 5'11" and weighs between 90 and 120 pounds, and the average male fashion model weighs between 120 and 160 pounds.

- Eating disorders are on the rise—in both women and men![5]

Having a positive attitude and accepting who you are is the first step to making healthy lifestyle changes. It is actually much easier to make permanent lifestyle changes once you accept the reality that you may never have a "perfect" body shape; the goal is good health and better living. Take a moment to jot down thoughts about your body image. What do you say to yourself? Are there societal attitudes or beliefs you've bought into? What needs to change in your thinking?

_____

_____

_____

_____

_____

A Redefinition of "Ideal"

The fashion industry is starting to wake up, and I'm glad to see it. The pressure is mounting to change the standards in the modeling world. Even magazines for fitness professionals are starting to use pictures of real bodies as they demonstrate the latest fitness trends—bodies that represent all shapes and sizes.

Success should come from how well you meet your goals for good health. Set your sights on healthy eating habits and regular physical activity, rather than comparing yourself to fashion magazines, actresses on TV, or even the scale for that matter.

Talk to your doctor, a nutritionist, or other health provider about what your ideal body weight should be. The goal is not to have a perfect model's figure but to live a healthier, happier and more productive life—in the body that you have! Don't make your goal unrealistic or unachievable. Even a 10 percent weight loss will result in improvements in your overall health and quality of life. There's a popular quote that goes something like this:

"Your body is where you will spend the rest of your life; isn't it about time you made it your home?" Actually, isn't it about time you made it God's home?

—See 1 Corinthians 6:19-20

WHERE DO I BEGIN? UNDERSTANDING THE TYPES OF CARDIOVASCULAR TRAINING

Often the hardest part of knowing where to begin is just that—knowing where to begin. There are hundreds of infomercials touting the praises of the latest workout craze. But if you are new to exercise, the thought of exercise can be intimidating.

Knowledge is power, and understanding the various types of exercise, especially cardiovascular exercise, can help you start on your new journey of health and wellness with power and confidence.

Cardiovascular exercises are designed to strengthen your heart and lungs and help you burn excess calories. But are they all the same?

TYPES OF CARDIOVASCULAR TRAINING

STEADY-STATE TRAINING (Aerobic) is a long and continuous workout in which the heart rate and oxygen consumption remain relatively stable. The intensity is defined as between 40 percent and 70 percent of your maximum heart rate. On an RPE chart, your efforts would fall between 4 and 6. This can be a good place for beginners to start as it is a great way to build endurance and can be done as low impact.

Steady-state exercise can offer "active recovery" after higher intensity days of exercise. By training your body to function for longer periods, your muscles will become more efficient at using oxygen, and your heart will get stronger. It also keeps you burning calories and breaking a sweat on those recovery days instead of completely taking a day off.

Examples of this style of workout would be brisk walking, swimming, jogging, water aerobics, dancing, aerobics, biking, and cardio machines.

ANAEROBIC TRAINING is fueled by energy stored in your muscles rather than relying on oxygen, such as in aerobic training. It consists of short, high-intensity bursts of activity that cause you to quickly get out of breath, such as sprinting, climbing a long flight of stairs, or heavy weight lifting. The benefits of anaerobic exercise are numerous. One benefit is that it builds and maintains lean muscle

MYplace O FOR FITNESS

mass. This increase in muscle mass and strength helps protect your joints, boosts metabolism, increases bone strength and density, and improves your energy.

INTERVAL TRAINING (IT) marries aerobic and anaerobic together to make powerful and effective exercise workouts. Interval training is easier than you might think. It simply alternates bursts of high-intensity periods with intervals of lower intensity or active rests. If you enjoy walking, you can achieve interval training by alternating walking with more intense periods of faster walking or jogging. I often use mailboxes or street signs as interval markers if I'm outdoors. With this type of training, you get all of the benefits of both steady-state and anaerobic together while saving yourself time.

The great thing about IT is that you get to set the pace. You determine the length and intensity of your intervals. Some days might be more intense than others depending on how you feel.

IT is not for everyone. If you have chronic conditions, you may want to discuss this type of workout with your doctor. However, recent studies have shown that short periods of interval training can be used safely in individuals with heart disease, type 2 diabetes, and obesity.

HIGH-INTENSITY INTERVAL TRAINING (HIIT) is a more intense form of IT (see "No Time to Work Out? Try HIIT"). The goal is to reach 80-95 percent of your maximum heart rate during the working phase of exercise. Tabata, 3-2-1, and Sprint are types of HIIT training.

Jim had a goal to lose 30 pounds. He was tracking his food but was confused about exercise, so he wasn't exercising at all. Knowing this was a big component of overall wellness, he wanted to know what he should do to accomplish his goal. First, we spent some time talking about various types of exercise. From there we developed an overall plan that included several different styles of exercise. He would alternate days of steady-state exercise with various interval training and strength training. With a focused exercise plan in hand, Jim felt confident to begin. He started to see results in just a few weeks. And after six months, Jim reached his goal.

During those six months, there were times when Jim hit plateaus. We'd make a few adjustments to his plan, and before we knew it, the scale would start to move again.

MY JOURNEY

With this knowledge in hand, ask yourself the following questions (taken from the American Council on Exercise Fit Facts):

A yes to any one of the following questions means you should talk with your doctor, by phone or in person, before you start an exercise program. Explain which questions you answered yes to and the activities you are planning to pursue.

1. Have you been told that you have a heart condition and should only participate in physical activity recommended by a doctor?

2. Do you feel pain (or discomfort) in your chest when you do physical activity? When you are not participating in physical activity? While at rest, do you frequently experience fast, irregular heartbeats or very slow beats?

3. Do you ever become dizzy and lose your balance, or lose consciousness? Have you fallen more than twice in the past year (no matter what the reason)?

4. Do you have a bone or joint problem that could worsen as a result of physical activity? Do you have pain in your legs or buttocks when you walk?

5. Do you take blood pressure or heart medications?

6. Do you have any cuts or wounds on your feet that don't seem to heal?

7. Have you experienced unexplained weight loss in the past six months?

8. Are you aware of any reason why you should not participate in physical activity?

9. Are you planning to engage in vigorous activities?

If you answered no to all of these questions, then you passed the first round of questions—you can be reasonably sure that you can safely take part in at least a moderate-intensity physical-activity program, such as steady-state exercise or moderate interval training.

If you are a man over 45 or a woman over 55 and want to exercise more vigorously, you should check with your physician before getting started.

I wish I were able to sit with you to develop a personalized plan, but I'm hoping that this book will give you all the information you need to do just that. As you

MYplace O FOR FITNESS

move through this book, underline what stands out to you, write notes to yourself in the margins—but most of all put it into action.

"Knowledge is of no value unless you put it into practice"

—Anton Chekhov

STRENGTH TRAINING 101

"He gives strength to the weary and increases the power of the weak"
—Isaiah 40:29

Strength training should be an exerciser's best friend. The benefits are so numerous. Yet, I can't count the number of times I've been asked if strength training really makes that much of a difference. The simple answer is yes! Just look at them all:

- Halts bone loss and builds bone density
- Improves balance, posture and stability
- Increases muscle tone and lean body mass
- Decreases or minimizes risk of osteoporosis
- Improves your overall flexibility by working muscles through a full range of motion
- Improves your body composition by reducing body fat and by gaining muscle
- Increases muscle endurance, strength and power which equal usable energy
- Increases HDL (good cholesterol) and decreases LDL (bad cholesterol)
- Reduces risk of diabetes
- Lowers risk of cardiovascular disease
- Lowers blood pressure
- Increases lung function
- Lowers risk of breast cancer (reduces high estrogen levels linked to the disease)

Talk to your doctor before you begin your program, especially if you have high blood pressure or other health problems.

MYplace O FOR FITNESS

- Reduces symptoms of PMS (Premenstrual Syndrome)

- Reduces stress and anxiety

- Increases endorphins; improves depression

- Decreases colds and illness

- Reduces likelihood of injury

- Allows you to fall asleep faster and sleep more deeply

- Increases self-confidence and self-image

- Increases digestion and elimination

- *And* weight loss!

Miriam Nelson, PhD, leading researcher and author of the Strong Women book series, believes that you can actually turn back the clock of aging by incorporating strength training into your exercise routine. She and her colleagues proved it after conducting several studies that took the medical community by surprise. One such study with postmenopausal women showed that "after one year of strength training, their bodies were 15 to 20 years more youthful."[7] The women showed gains in their bone density, traded fat for muscle, looked trimmer, and dropped a size or two. Other studies done on men, nursing home residents, and people aged 35 to 90 have shown similar results.[8] Who wouldn't want that?

I'm always blessed when I have students come to class who have been sent there by their doctor. I love that the doctor understands its importance and that the patient listened to their doctor. Take Jenny, for example, who at 70 listened when her doctor told her she needed to strength train; so she joined my class with her friend. Jenny is a walker who has osteopenia (a precursor to osteoporosis). Jenny already knew the value of exercise, so when her doctor explained all the benefits of strength training, it wasn't hard for her to accept her doctor's advice.

I also love seeing the joy students find as they incorporate strength training into their routine and see themselves growing stronger. It blesses me to hear their reports on how they are able to handle everyday tasks more effectively. Laura shared with me the increase in energy and stamina she's experiencing as she works full time and cares for her disabled son. Christie told me how she's been able to handle harder gardening tasks, such as hauling mulch, more easily than before. And the list goes on: my friend Carole, at 75, is still lifting 12, 15, and 25 pound weights so that she can stay strong to play with grandchildren and great-grand-children.

Yet, I also see others who go through the motions of strength training but simply aren't getting all they can from it. The biggest culprit is growing comfortable with the size of the weights they are using.

These three factors will determine what you get out of your strength-training workouts:

1. The size of the weights or the amount of resistance used

2. The number of reps you are using

3. The speed of each movement*

(*There is a difference in training for strength rather than endurance. Both are important. When training for strength use slower movements and heavier weights or stronger resistance bands. Training for endurance uses slightly lighter weights working at a faster pace with a larger number of sets.)

Note: Women have different hormone levels than men. You simply won't bulk up like a man—find definition yes, bulk no.

WHAT YOU NEED TO GET STARTED

Handheld Weights

Going to the store to choose weights can be intimidating. You want to select weights that are heavy enough to be challenging and take the muscle to "failure" (meaning that you can't do another rep using proper form).

A good way to determine what weight size is right for you is to perform bicep curls in the store. Hold the weights slightly in front of you at waist level so that your arms are at a 90-degree angle. Don't rest your elbows on your waist; keep them in front of your body. The palms of your hands should be facing up as you hold the weights. Slowly lift the weights toward your chest in a count of 1, 2, 3, 4 and release in 1, 2 back to waist level. If you cannot perform 8 repetitions, then the weights are too heavy. If you can easily perform 8 repetitions or more, then the weights are too light. Strive for weights that are difficult but allow you to maintain good form while lifting through the repetitions.

DIY—Don't have the money to purchase weights? Go to your cupboard or pantry. Many everyday items that you purchase from the grocery store will work for you. A 16 oz can weighs one pound. A liter of soda weighs 2.2 pounds. A gallon of water weighs 8.3 pounds. See how you can progress using common pantry items?

Resistance Bands

Resistance bands or tubes are made of elastic or rubber tubing. Most fitness stores have them available in several resistances. Try them out at the store to make sure you purchase the right one for you. You should be able to move through the whole range of motion of each exercise. If you can't perform the full range of motion, then you need a lighter resistance until you can work up to a heavier load. Bands and tubes can be very effective for strength cross-training because they challenge muscle groups in different ways than hand weights. When you use bands or tubes, always make sure you control them as you move through each exercise slowly and in a controlled manner as the band or tube provides external resistance. You should always start with the band or tube in a taut position, pull out through the range of motion, and return to a taut position. Never let the band or tube sag as you release the motion.

Body-weight Strength Training

Many of the popular workouts these days (P90X, Insanity, HIIT classes) use body-weight exercises to incorporate strength training. Using your own body weight to train requires nothing but you. How great is that? The best part is that all you need is a floor, which makes exercising at home a breeze. Planks, mountain climbers, burpees, bear walks, inchworms, wall sits, tricep dips, and lunges are just a few examples. (Don't let the names scare you—there are modifications for all of these!)

Keys to Proper Strength Training

Keep a tight core. My students often tell me that they hear me saying these words when they are exercising on their own outside of class. Torso stabilization and good

MY JOURNEY

posture are key to proper alignment and execution of most strength-training movements. Look in the mirror and check your posture with the following:

- Neck is in line with the spine.

- Shoulders are back, down, and relaxed.

- Back is straight.

- Abdominal muscles are tightened.

- Gluteal muscles are tightened; pelvis is slightly tucked under.

- Knees are soft, not locked or bent.

Stop when you have performed all the reps you can do using proper form. Bad posture indicates fatigue. Don't compromise your position or you risk injury.

Avoid hyperextension and locking joints, especially your elbows and knees. If you lock a joint, that joint (and not the muscles) is holding the weight, which leaves you vulnerable to injury by stressing the joint.

Keep all movements slow and controlled. Don't rush through any of the movements. Avoid heaving the weight and having to brake it at the end of the range of motion.

Remember to breathe. Exhale on exertion (when you are moving against gravity), and inhale on the release. This is one of the most common mistakes. Holding your breath can raise blood pressure.

Strength train at least two times per week. Once a week isn't enough to see change. Three times a week can be even more effective. Always leave one day of rest between strength-training workouts so that your muscles can recover. The amount of time for each session will vary and will depend on the number of muscle groups worked. Usually, a 30-minute session will provide enough time to target each muscle group.

Keep in mind that the "use it or lose it" rule is real. Strength is lost quickly when you stop doing strength training (in other words, your muscles will atrophy). If you experience illness or take time off for vacation or holidays, you may have to build back up. So, start back at a lighter weight rather than picking up where you left off.

myplace ○ FOR FITNESS

"Love the Lord your God with all your heart and with all your soul and with all your strength"
—Deuteronomy 6:5

STRENGTH TRAINING GUIDE AND WORKOUT

Start with 8-10 repetitions to equal 1 set. Work up to 3 sets. Using 3 to 5lb weights, increase the weight as sets become easier. Set a goal to get to 8lbs or higher.

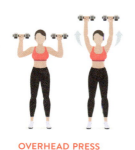

OVERHEAD PRESS

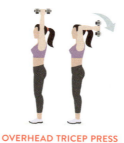

OVERHEAD TRICEP PRESS

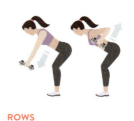

ROWS

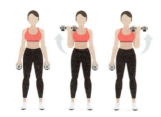

STANDING ALTERNATING BICEP CURL OR SEATED BICEP CURL

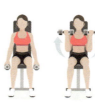

MY JOURNEY

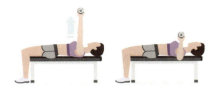

CHEST PRESS OR PUSH UPS

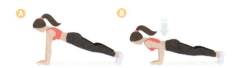

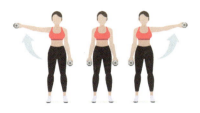

ALTERNATING LATERAL RISES

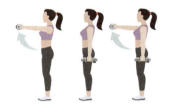

ALTERNATING FRONT RISES

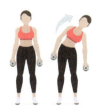

STANDING SIDE LEANS W/ WEIGHTS

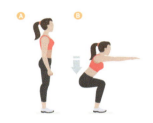

SQUATS

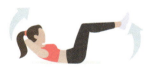

ABDOMINAL CRUNCHES

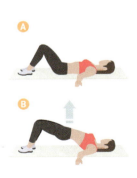

BRIDGES

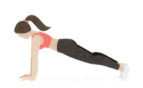

PLANK HOLD

83

FLEXIBILITY AND BALANCE TRAINING

My husband and daughter are not naturally limber. While I can bend forward and touch my toes with ease, my husband is lucky if he can manage to reach his knees. When my daughter was 3 or 4 years old, I took her to a toddler dance and tumbling class. After a couple of weeks, the teacher actually suggested another class for her to take due to her lack of flexibility. Throughout her childhood, when it came time for the Presidential Fitness Challenge at school, she would excel in all of the exercises (including pull-ups) with one exception—the V-sit reach. She simply was built with tighter muscles and ligaments. Today her focus is on workouts that increase her range of motion because she knows it's importance to her overall health.

Flexibility and balance should be an integral part of everyone's health and wellness plan. If it's a struggle for you, know that with consistent training both will improve.

Flexibility, or stretching, exercises are one of the quickest ways to increase your fitness level. Many medical conditions, such as arthritis, fibromyalgia, or chronic joint pain, can all experience positive benefits from this type of training, including the following:

- Promotion and maintenance of range of motion in joints

- Improvement of posture

- Enhancement of physical and mental relaxation

- Release of muscle tension and soreness

- Reduction of risk of injury

As in the case of my husband and daughter, your flexibility is primarily tied to your genetics. However, gender, age, level of physical activity, and medical condition also play a big part. Studies show that most loss of flexibility and balance is a result of inactivity rather than the aging process. The less active we are, the less flexible we are likely to be.

I once watched a video of a doctor stricken with arthritis who was bound to a wheelchair. Not being content with this, he decided to develop a stretching program for himself. He started with a simple piece of PVC piping. He would take the piping in both hands and raise his hands over his head. Then he would do some torso rotations. Before you knew it, he had built stretching exercise structures using this piping, that allowed him to develop strength and flexibility in more parts of his body. The last part of the video showed him walking freely, no longer needing the wheelchair. I was convinced. Movement is critical, and flexibility exercises and stretching are as important as any other type of exercise.

Stretching and Flexibility Basics

1. Warm up your muscles before beginning any workout. No longer is static stretching used during a warm-up. The new rule of thumb is to warm up using dynamic movements. These are movements that mimic the type of exercise, sport, or activity you'll be doing. For example, professional soccer players will often be seen before a game moving across the field using hip internal and external rotations to warm up the hips, or straight-leg kicks to warm up the hamstrings, both being essential to the type of movement they'll be doing.

2. Do stretch after a workout. This is where static stretching is excellent and can help improve range. Be sure to keep it gentle. Feeling tension when you stretch is normal, but pain means you've gone too far.

3. Try not to hold your breath. Breathe freely and relaxed as you stretch.

4. During static stretching, hold each stretch for 30 seconds; then release the stretch slightly for just a second and then move back into the stretch. This should allow you to be able to move deeper into the stretch.

5. Don't bounce during a static stretch. This type of stretching is called ballistic stretching and can stretch your muscles too fast and too far resulting in injury.

Balance and Stability Exercises (Base Training)

Falls, especially in older adults, are the number one reason for hip fractures. Stability and balance training begins by working your muscles in an unbalanced environment. Performing a one-legged squat, for example, causes your core to activate, strengthens the leg all the way from the quadricep to the ankle and foot, and results in improved balance and stability. Bosu balls are designed specifically for this type of training.

MYplace O FOR FITNESS

Many of us have adopted movement compensations that deactivate our core muscles, such as lower back, pelvis, hips and abdomen—movements such as favoring one side whi e standing (baby on the hip), walking or even sitting. This can come from weakness in any of the core muscles, with the result being poor posture or low-back pain.

Your core muscles provide the support system for almost any activity or motion your body engages in. A Harvard Medical School publication, *The Real-World Benefits of Strengthening Your Core*, states that "no matter where motion starts, it ripples upward and downward to adjoining links of the chain. Thus, weak or inflexible core muscles can impair how well your arms and legs function. And that saps power from many of the moves you make. A strong core also enhances balance and stability. Thus, it can help prevent falls and injuries during sports or other activities. In fact, a strong, flexible core underpins almost everything you do:

- O Everyday acts. Bending to put on shoes or scoop up a package, turning to look behind you, sitting in a chair, or simply standing still—these are just a few of the many mundane actions that rely on your core and that you might not notice until they become difficult or painful. Even basic activities of daily living—bathing or dressing, for example—call on your core.

- O On-the-job tasks. Jobs that involve lifting, twisting, and standing all rely on core muscles. But less obvious tasks—like sitting at your desk for hours—engage your core as well. Phone calls, typing, computer use, and similar work can make back muscles surprisingly stiff and sore, particularly if you're not strong enough to practice good posture and aren't taking sufficient breaks.

- O A healthy back. Low back pain—a debilitating, sometimes excruciating problem affecting four out of five Americans at some point in their lives—may be prevented by exercises that promote well-balanced, resilient core muscles. When back pain strikes, a regimen of core exercises is often prescribed to relieve it, coupled with medications, physical therapy, or other treatments if necessary.

- O Sports and other pleasurable activities. Golfing, tennis or other racquet sports, biking, running, swimming, baseball, volleyball, kayaking, rowing and many other athletic activities are powered by a strong core. Less often mentioned are sexual activities, which call for core power and flexibility, too.

MY JOURNEY

- **Housework, fix-it work, and gardening.** Bending, lifting, twisting, carrying, hammering, reaching overhead—even vacuuming, mopping, and dusting are acts that spring from, or pass through, the core.

- **Balance and stability.** Your core stabilizes your body, allowing you to move in any direction, even on the bumpiest terrain, or stand in one spot without losing your balance. Viewed this way, core exercises can lessen your risk of falling.

- **Good posture.** Weak core muscles contribute to slouching. Good posture trims your silhouette and projects confidence. More importantly, it lessens wear and tear on the spine and allows you to breathe deeply. Good posture helps you gain full benefits from the effort you put into exercising, too."

Yoga, Pilates, tai chi, stability balls, Bosu balls, balance boards, or just standing on one leg, all offer the benefit of forcing your body to stabilize itself. If the spiritual components of yoga or tai chi cause you pause, look for classes where this emphasis has been removed or replaced with a Christian emphasis. Praise Moves and Holy Yoga are two programs that bring a Christ-centered perspective to the workout.

Static stretching is something you can do when you are not getting ready for activity. If you've been sitting too long at work, or are just getting out of bed, taking time to stretch your muscles using static stretching will relieve stress and help prevent injuries, especially those nagging aches and pains that never seem to go away. Before you start though, take a minute to warm up. Do some marching in place or high knees; side-steps with arm circles are a good way to get the blood flowing.

Don't be discouraged by a limited range of motion due to excess body fat. Just keep at it. As you continue on your wellness journey, your body fat will decrease, and your flexibility will increase.

MYplace O FOR FITNESS

STRETCHING EXERCISES

NECK FLEXION EXTENSION STRETCH
(forward, then back)

NECK LATERAL FLEXION STRETCH
(one side, then the other)

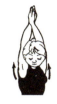

LATISSIMUS DORIS AND POSTERIOR DELTID STRETCH
(link hands, push elbows together)

TRICEPS STRETCH
(pulll elbow across and down)

SHOULDER ROTATOR STRETCH
(using towel, pull up with the top arm then down with the other)

PECTORAL STRETCH AT 90° AND 120°
(use a doorway or post)

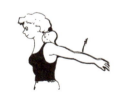

BICEP STRETCH
(hands apart)

SUPRASPINATUS STRETCH
(keep elbow parallel to ground)

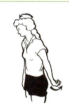

WRIST EXTENSOR STRETCH
(tilt head to opposite side, keep elbow straight)

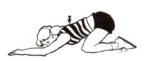

THORACIC EXTENSION STRETCH
(reach forward with arms, push chest towards flood, arch back down, backside behind knees)

LATERAL FLEXION STRETCH
(one side, then the other, push pelvis across as you bend)

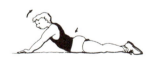

LUMBAR EXTENSION AND ABDOMINAL STRETCH
(be gentle if sore)

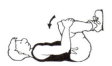

LUMBAR FLEXION STRECH
(be gentle if sore)

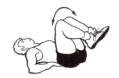

LUMBAR ROTATION STRETCH
(rotate legs one side, then the other side, draw in and brace stomach muscles at the same time, breathe)

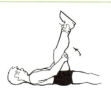

HAMSTRING STRETCH
(straighten leg—with foot pointed and with foot pulled back towards the knee)

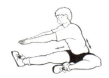

HAMSTRING STRETCH
(commence with knee slightly bent, then push knee straight as tension allows, push chest towards foot)

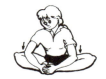

ABDUCTOR STRETCH
(push down with elbows on knees very gently, keep back straight)

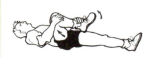

GLUTEAL STRETCH
(pull knee and lower leg towards opposite shoulder)

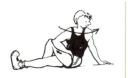

GLUTEAL AND LUMBAR ROTATION STRETCH
(hands apart)

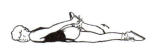

QUADRICEPS STRETCH
(keep pelvis on floor)

QUADRICEPS STRETCH

ABDUCTOR STRETCH
(keep foot pointing forward, lunge sideways on bent knee, keep back straight)

HIP FLEXOR STRETCH
(keep back straight, tuck bottom under, lunge forward on front leg)

TENSOR FASCIA STRETCH
(continue to push bottom forward, whilst pushing hip to the side)

GASTROCNEMIUS STRETCH
(keep knee straight and heel down, feet facing forward)

5 FITNESS MYTHS WE NEED TO LET GO OF

Here are five myths about fitness that we have all believed at one time or another.

I know I'm working hard if I sweat a lot.
Remember when I said that I used to believe this? It simply isn't true. People sweat at different rates, so sweating isn't a true indicator of a hard workout. Use the tools provided in the "Know Your Fitness Numbers" section to truly be able to gauge your workout effectiveness. Working in your target heart rate zone is a better guide than how much you are sweating.

I can eat whatever I want after a hard workout.
Oh, how we all want this one to be true, but unfortunately it isn't. Many people underestimate the calories they consume and overestimate the number of calories they burn during a workout, according to a 2010 study published in the Journal of Sports Medicine & Physical Fitness. Make sure you track your calories and stay on goal. A stop by the coffee shop after a workout can undo all of your efforts.

Soreness equals a hard workout.
While it's not uncommon to feel some delayed onset muscle soreness (DOMS) after a workout session, your goal shouldn't be soreness. It should be getting healthy and fit and strong. Consider using a foam roller or tennis ball to massage any tender areas. Overtraining and lack of recovery time can lead to injury. If you are still feeling soreness after a few days, you may need to evaluate whether you are overtraining or have an injury. Pain is different from soreness and could be a sign of injury. Sharp pain while performing an exercise means stop—don't continue!

Crunches will flatten my abs.
While we all want that smooth flat stomach, surprisingly, crunches may not get you there. To lose weight from your midsection requires fat burning. Try a HIIT or interval training program that incorporates body-weight exercises that target the full core, such as mountain climbers, squats, planks and bridges.

You need to do static stretching before a workout.

While it's true that a good warm-up is essential to any workout, dynamic stretching is where it's at. Dynamic stretching, or dynamic warm-up, is where you practice the movements you'll be using during your workout. This prepares your body for the work you'll be doing and increases your range of motion. Save the static stretching for your post-workout stretch.

MYplace O FOR FITNESS

ACTIVITY TRACKER—DO I REALLY NEED ONE?

The simple answer is no. Being fit does not depend on wearing a tracker or using an app; however, if you are like me, you might find just the right motivation using one.

Here are some questions to consider when answering this question:

o Do you like data, numbers and facts?

o Do you like competition? Wearing a tracker might give you the extra incentive to move more—and prove that you did it.

o Do you feel like you hit a lot of roadblocks? A tracker could be just the thing to help push you through when you seem to have reached a plateau. With a tracker, you can easily look back over the week to see how you did in accomplishing your activity goals.

Which One Is the Best?
The simple answer is that there is no one tracker that's best for everyone. Personal style, preferences, and budgets all play a part in your decision. It might be that your cell phone determines which tracker works best for you. The Apple Watch, for example, works only with an iPhone. So, while it's a top pick among trainers, it won't be right for you if you don't use an iPhone.

If you use an online tool for tracking your meals, that online tool may only link to specific trackers. Check out the FAQ section on tracker websites to see what each tracker is most compatible to.

What Features Most Interest You?
Do you have specific goals in mind for using the tracker, or are you just tracking steps? Knowing what your goals are will help you determine what trackers are best to help you meet those goals. If all you are interested in is tracking your daily steps, then an inexpensive pedometer might be the best way to go.

Knowing which tracker offers what features is key. Just because a tracker is expensive doesn't mean it will offer you the features you are looking for. Do your research before you buy. Make sure you are getting all the features you are looking for. If, for example, you are looking to run a 5K, make sure you have a tracker that allows you to compare your daily, weekly, and even monthly data.

Do Trackers Automatically Know When I'm Working Out?

Maybe. Most trackers record your activities of daily living, such as walking around, getting up and down, or climbing stairs; however, not all have an automatic launch feature that detects when you begin a workout. You may have to manually launch your workout from your tracker or phone. When you manually launch your tracker, it will collect data, such as heart rate, calorie burn, pace, and distance, just to name a few, that will give you important information as you move toward your goal. Just don't forget to stop the workout function on your tracker when you are finished.

Are Trackers Accurate?

Maybe. It depends on what you are looking at. An ACE-commissioned study done in 2015 showed that most trackers are accurate when counting steps but less so when considering agility drills. If you are doing strength training, for example, a tracker might not accurately reflect your activity level. That's where additional features, such as heart rate monitoring, can be beneficial. Also, technology is changing constantly. As technology improves, so too does accuracy.

The bottom line is this: Will having a tracker motivate you toward a lifestyle of activity and wellness? If the answer to that is yes, then run to your nearest store and buy one!

NO TIME TO WORK OUT? TRY HIIT

Who says your workout has to last one hour? What if you could burn more calories and fat in shorter amounts of time, boost your metabolism, do a workout that requires no equipment, and has anti-aging properties? Would you do it? I would and I do!

Have you ever heard of **HIIT**? The acronym stands for High-Intensity Interval Training and it's one of the hottest new fitness trends around. For good reason! The benefits are many and the rewards are great.

The truth is that HIIT has been used for years by professional athletes. Two of the very first pioneers of the HIIT training method were speed-skating coaches for the 1990 Japanese Olympic team. They had an unusual training technique that used short but intense bursts of effort followed by an even shorter rest period. The results were increased short-term explosive strength, which is needed in speed skating, but they also found it to increase long-term endurance, also needed in speed skating. And the rest, as they say, is history. Now athletes worldwide in just about every sport use this type of training—and so can you. Even the most sedentary person can benefit from using this type of training. Veteran exercisers use HIIT to find new challenges, and beginner exercisers can use it to see results more quickly.

HIIT is short bursts of strenuous exercise intermingled with brief periods of rest. There are many different formats of HIIT. Tabata training is one where you do 20 seconds of intense work (90-95 percent) followed by 10 seconds of complete rest. Repeat this for 8 rounds and rest for 1 minute. When done at the highest level, you can do one Tabata set (4 minutes) and be done. When using this method at a lower level, say 80-85 percent, add additional sets to make it a 20-minute workout.

Another variety of HIIT is One-to-One. Choose 30 seconds, 45 seconds, or 1 minute. This becomes both your work and your rest time. Let's use jumping jacks as an example. Perform the jacks for 30 seconds and then rest for 30 seconds. Repeat the sequence for 10 rounds. If variety is what you need, change the exercises every two rounds as you move through the workout. After the 10 rounds, take a longer rest and then repeat another set.

A popular HIIT routine with celebrities is 3-2-1, which stands for 3 minutes of cardio, 2 minutes of strength or resistance training, and 1 minute of core exercise.

You can do all the cardio at once, varying the intensity from low to high, and then follow that with strength, and then core. Or you can mix it up by doing cardio 1, strength 1, cardio 2, strength 2, cardio 3 and core—all performed using 1-minute intervals. Then rest for 2 minutes. This is where creativity can come into play. You can use the same exercise throughout each segment, for example: cardio—all jumping jacks; strength—all military press; core—all abdominal crunches. Or you can mix it up: cardio—1 minute of jacks, 1 minute of mountain climbers, and 1 minute of squat jumps; strength—1 minute of military press, 1 minute of bent rows; core—1 minute of Russian twists, 1 minute of abdominal crunches.

Some people like to add more sets in, making it 5-4-3-2-1. Choose 5 exercises performed for 1 minute, then rest 1 minute. Then four exercises, and rest; 3 exercises, and rest; 2 exercises, and rest; and finish with one last one.

Any cardio activity you enjoy, such as running, biking, swimming, rowing, jumping rope, can be turned into a HIIT routine by increasing your intensity and adding in rests. Let's take running as an example. Always start with a dynamic warm-up of 2 to 6 minutes depending on your activity. In this case it's running, so start by walking at a good pace for 1 minute, jog lightly for 1 minute, and then repeat each. You are warmed up and ready to move into HIIT. Using the One-to-One method, jog lightly for 30 seconds, then pick up the pace for 30 seconds, move back to jogging lightly for 30 seconds, etc. Repeat for 10 rounds and then walk, allowing yourself to rest for 2 minutes. You are either finished with your workout or you can repeat it for a second set. Do you see how this can work with just about any type of activity?

With HIIT you are constantly pushing yourself out of your comfort zone, which keeps your workout from getting boring! That's the great thing about HIIT—the variety. You're probably asking, "Which HIIT workout is best?" They all are—meaning they all offer the same results. So, do a few of them and find the one you enjoy most.

I teach the Tabata method at the gym. I enjoy it the most; however, I also like 3-2-1 and One-to-One and will add them in for variety.

Just the name alone tells you that this workout is going to require more intensity than a casual stroll down the street—*High Intensity*. Using the Rate of Perceived Exertion table (RPE), you should work at an intensity rate of 8 or above on a scale of 1-10. You want to work hard enough that it is difficult to carry on a conversation. If you are able to carry on a conversation with a friend or exercise buddy, then you aren't working hard enough. Knowing your personal fitness numbers will help you determine your personal workout intensity and goals. (See "Know Your Fitness Numbers" and the Rate of Perceived Exertion table.)

During steady-state training, your heart rate stays at roughly 50 percent to 80 percent of your maximum heart rate, keeping it steady. Examples of this include jogging outdoors or on a treadmill at a consistent pace, pedaling a stationary exercise bike without changing resistance or speeds, or any cardio that uses mostly the same intensity throughout a class. However, you can turn any steady-state workout into a HIIT workout by simply increasing the intensity to over 80 percent of your maximum heart rate and by using short bursts followed by brief rests.

I could list study after study that has proven HIIT workouts to be more effective than steady-state cardio when it comes to burning fat. Dr. Martin Gibala is a physiologist and leading researcher on HIIT from Canada's McMaster University. He likened HIIT to the way kids play on the playground. They start and stop, sprint, skip and jump. They don't run at steady paces doing only one thing. They swing from monkey bars and then chase each other. It's a very natural way to play and to be active, which may be one reason HIIT is so enjoyable and good for us, according to Dr. Gibala. It's inherent in us.

In one of many studies, Dr. Gibala and his team divided their study participants into two teams. One did 20 weeks of traditional aerobics and the other did 15 weeks of HIIT. While the first group burned 48 more calories per exercise session than the HIIT group—are you ready for this?—the HIIT group burned 900 percent more fat in the 15 weeks than the first group burned in 20 weeks. Nine hundred percent more fat burned! That's amazing—astonishing really.

The reason for this fat burn is simple: it's what happens once your workout is over.

Your body has to work extra hard to return your systems to normal—your body temperature, heart rate, and blood pressure, to name a few. This requires extra calories, which is the EPOC effect. EPOC stands for excess post-exercise oxygen consumption and it is the reason the HIIT workout can be short and effective. So, for hours after a HIIT workout, your body is on fire burning up that extra fuel.

Another recent Dr. Gibala study looked at the benefits of adding a single minute (60 seconds broken into three 20-second intervals) within a 10-minute workout of intense cycling three times a week. They compared the results to a 45-minute steady-state cycling workout. At the end of the study, the steady-state group had cycled for 27 hours and the HIIT group only 6 hours. The results showed virtually the same gains physiologically in the two groups. It doesn't take long to decide which you'd prefer—27 hours or 6?

Speaking of long term, HIIT has also been shown to improve glucose tolerance, and blood sugar regulation in type 2 diabetics, and even to increase the function of our mitochondria, which are our cells' energy powerhouses, allowing us to fuel our body more efficiently.

Because of their intensity, HIIT workouts are more exhaustive and require longer rest periods in between workouts, whereas steady-state training can be done daily. A good rule of thumb is to alternate days of HIIT with steady-state training to allow for recovery.

10 Reasons to Do HIIT

1. You can do HIIT anywhere—inside or outside.

2. It improves heart health.

3. It improves blood sugar regulation.

4. You don't need any special equipment.

5. You can do HIIT with friends or all by yourself.

6. HIIT is extremely efficient on time.

7. HIIT challenges you both mentally and physically.

8. It's a great way to burn fat while maintaining muscle mass.

9. HIIT is a great way to increase your metabolism and burn calories long after your workout is over.

10. HIIT is anti-aging!

Wait! What? Anti-aging? Yes, you bet it is. Mayo Clinic researchers have discovered another amazing benefit. Its anti-aging benefits. Remember those cellular powerhouses? A study conducted through a Mayo research team found that HIIT has tremendous impact on our mitochondria, which tend to deteriorate as we age. Keeping mitochondria healthy can reverse some signs of age-related decline within cells, say the researchers. The team studied two groups of sedentary adults, one group aged 18-30 and one group aged 65-80, and found that HIIT got the biggest benefit at the cellular level over a strength-training workout and a combined workout of cardio (cycling) and strength. The younger age group experienced a 49 percent boost in mitochondrial capacity, while the older age group saw a whopping 69 percent increase!

While research shows a direct correlation between physical activity and life expectancy, it also shows that HIIT can activate telomerase, a well-known anti-aging enzyme in our bodies that lengthens telomeres. Telomeres allow cells to divide without losing genes. This is necessary for growing new skin, blood, bone, and other cells, and researchers believe that longer telomeres lengthen our lifespans.

As they say on TV: But wait, there's more! HIIT's anti-aging benefits also include:

1. Firmer skin/fewer wrinkles

2. Increased energy

3. Boosted metabolism

4. Improved libido

5. Muscle tone improvement

6. Reduced body fat

Who doesn't want all of those benefits?

In addition to all of the above, one of the most important benefits of HIIT is that it can help balance the hormones that are responsible for weight gain and some of our unhealthy eating habits. Three hormones, ghrelin, leptin, and testosterone, are all affected by HIIT.

When you think of ghrelin, think "grrrrrr." Known as the "hunger hormone," it's what causes the munchies, or your cravings for sweet, salty and fried foods. Produced in the stomach, ghrelin is believed to be the only hormone that stimulates appetite and is released in response to stressful situations. Ever wonder why you want to eat when you get stressed? Thank ghrelin. Fortunately, HIIT decreases ghrelin levels.

Leptin is the hormone produced by the fat cells in our bodies and is known as the "starvation hormone." Its main role is to regulate how many calories we eat and burn, and how much fat we carry on our bodies. Thermogenesis, a process that makes heat, particularly in the muscles, regulates the number of calories you burn. Thermogenesis is substantially increased by the hormone leptin, helping you to burn fat. As leptin rises, your appetite decreases; and as leptin falls, your appetite increases. When you eat too much (past that feeling of being full), don't get enough sleep, deal with too much stress, and/or don't exercise, your body can ignore the leptin signal, causing you to develop leptin resistance. When you become leptin resistant, your body isn't able to stimulate your metabolism or suppress your appetite. The result is weight gain. And that's where HIIT comes in. HIIT increases leptin levels. In fact, research continues to show that HIIT actually balances both leptin and ghrelin, which increases your fat burning and weight loss.

Then there is testosterone. Testosterone naturally decreases as we age. HIIT keeps testosterone levels strong, which keeps you strong and burning fat. All humans have testosterone, but men have more than women, which is why men bulk up but women don't. Let's just break that myth right now: women just simply don't have enough testosterone in our bodies to allow that to happen. Because HIIT often uses body-weight exercises, you can get the benefit of strength training without having to lift weights.

The news keeps getting better. Typically, exercising can cause leptin and testosterone to counteract each other, negating the positive benefits of both, which can leave one frustrated and gaining weight. However, according to a study published in the journal *Endocrine*, HIIT workouts encourage a very unique situation where leptin and testosterone work well together, leaving you with the benefits of *both* weight-loss-producing hormones!

As with any activity, you want to maximize the effectiveness of HIIT. Research, such as a study published in the Journal of Physiology, shows that exercising first thing in the morning controls ghrelin and leptin, and exercising on an empty stomach improves glucose tolerance and insulin sensitivity, contributing both to the prevention of type 2 diabetes and to increased weight loss.

MYplace ○ FOR FITNESS

I recommend doing the following:

1. Consult your doctor to make sure this is the right exercise for you.

2. Add in one HIIT workout to your already existing exercise program.

3. Rest in between HIIT workouts.

4. As you see improvement, add in one or two additional HIIT workouts.

5. Vary your HIIT workouts.

6. Modify as necessary.

TYPE	SETS	DURATION
TABATA	8	4 minutes
ONE-TO-ONE	10	10 minutes
3-2-1	5	30 minutes
TEMPO	AMRAP	10 minutes
SPRINT	4-6	18-27 minutes
SHORT SPRINT	60	20 minutes

MY JOURNEY

WORK / REST INTERVALS	BENEFIT / EXAMPLES
20 sec / 10 sec	Popular, improves conditioning, burns more calories in 4 min., requires all-out effort
30 sec / 30 sec	Easy to perform and adapt to variety of fitness levels by increasing the work or decreasing the rest
3 min, 2 min, 1 min / 30 sec	Popular with celebrities, quick workout with big results. Start with cardio 1 / strength 1, cardio 2 / strength 2, cardio 3, core 1 or 3 min cardio (alternating hi/lo), 2 min strength, 1 min core
80% effort / active rest	Example: Sprinting up a flight of stairs, walking back down
30 sec / 4 min	Challenging at 100% effort, rest is long for recovery and to achieve conditioning results
30 sec / 30 sec	Less demanding, effective for conditioning and fat loss

HIIT CIRCUIT WORKOUTS

- Perform each exercise for 30 secs with 10 seconds rest in between.
- Rest for 2 minutes between each full circuit. Work up to repeating the circuit twice.
- All exercises can be modified for various exercise levels and abilities.

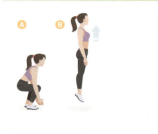

SQUAT JUMPS

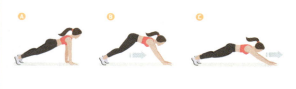

WALKOUTS OR INCH WORMS

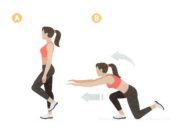

SKATERS

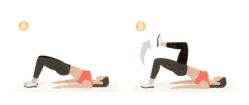

BRIDGE WALKS

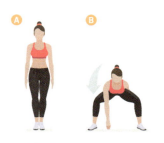

POWER SQUAT TOUCH

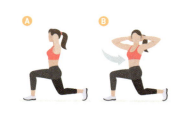

LUNGE WITH TORSO ROTATION

MY JOURNEY

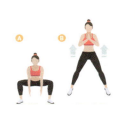

PILE JUMPS

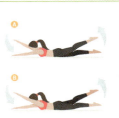

SWIMMING

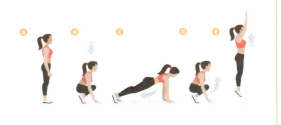

BURPEES

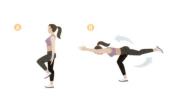

AIRPLANES

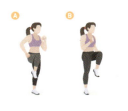

HIGH KNEES

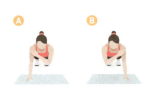

PLANK SHOULDER TAPS

HIIT CIRCUIT WORKOUTS

- Perform each exercise for 30 sec.

- After each exercise alternate a cardio exercise such as jumping jacks, squat jumps, mountain climbers, burpees, high knees.

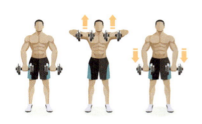

UPRIGHT ROW

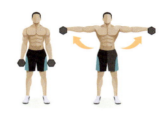

LATERAL RAISE

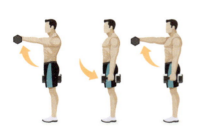

FRONT RAISE

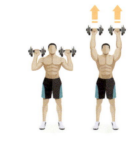

MILITARY PRESS

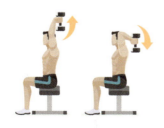

OVERHEAD TRCEP PRESS

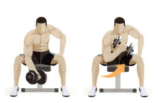

BICEP PRESS

MY JOURNEY

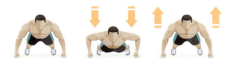

PUSH UPS

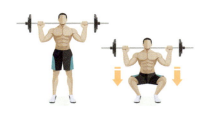

SQUAT WITH OR WITHOUT WEIGHTS

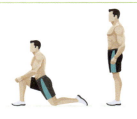

LUNGES WITH OR WITHOUT WEIGHTS

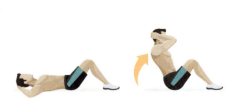

ABDOMINAL CRUNCHES

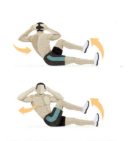

ABDOMINAL ROTATIONS

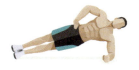

SIDE PLANK
HOLD FOR 30 SEC RIGHT AND LEFT

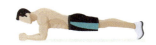

PLANK
START AT 30 SEC WORKING UP TO 2 MIN

MYplace O FOR FITNESS

WATER: THE EVERYDAY GUZZLE

Water—we literally can't live without it. The average human body is 75 percent water. Our bodies need it to regulate our body temperature, protect vital organs, lubricate our joints, help our digestive system, and transport nutrients to our cells. Getting even a little dehydrated can throw off a body's delicate balance. Our brains and muscles are each made of 75 percent water, with bones containing 22 percent. Read the following list to see how not drinking enough water can literally make you sick:

- Fatigue
- High blood pressure
- Allergies and asthma
- Skin disorders
- High cholesterol
- Kidney or bladder problems
- Digestive disorders
- Constipation
- Joint stiffness or pain
- Weight gain
- Premature aging

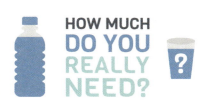

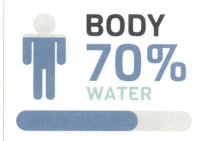

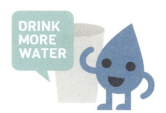

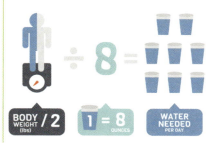

MY JOURNEY

WATER

DEHYDRATION - WHY IT'S MAKING YOU FAT AND SICK?

SKIN DISORDERS Dehydration impairs the elimination of toxins through High Cholesterol When the body is dehydrated it will produce more cholesterol to prevent water loss from the cells. This makes your skin more vulnerable to skin disorders such as dermatitis, psoriasis, wrinkling and discoloration.

FATIGUE Dehydration causes the enzymatic activity in the body to slow down, resulting in tiredness and fatigue.

HIGH BLOOD PRESSURE When dehydrated blood becomes thicker causing resistance to blood flow resulting in elevated blood pressure.

ASTHMA & ALLERGIES Deydration results in your airways restricting in order to conserve water. The more water you lose the more histamine increases.

BLADDER OR KIDNEY PROBLEMS The body is more prone to infection, inflammation and pain when dehydrated due to accumulated toxins and acid that provide the perfect environment for bacteria to thrive.

CONSTIPATION & DIGESTIVE PROBLEMS The colon is one of the primary regions the body draws water from in order to provide fluids or other critical body functions. Dehydratiorn slows waste elimination whichh leads to constipation and other digestive disorders such as ulcers, gastritis and acid reflux.

JOINT PAIN OR STIFFNESS All joints have cartilage padding which is composed mainly of water. When the body is dehydrated, cartilage is weakened and joint repair is slow.

WEIGHT GAIN The body, when dehydrated, stores toxins in fat cells instead of eliminating them In order for the body to release fat it needs to be sufficiently remove the toxins.

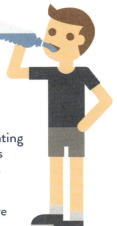

On average you should aim to drink 6-8 ounces of water every day.

Breathing, sweating, urinating and eliminating waste results in a loss of about 10 cups of water per day for the average adult.

Exercise, illness, pregnancy and breastfeeding are all factors that require increased water consumption.

MYplace **O** FOR FITNESS

So, when it comes to exercise, do you know how much water you need? Each of us is different. Our sweat rate, length and intensity of workout, along with the atmosphere we exercise in, are all important factors to consider when determining our needs.

"Your ability to perform athletically can decline with a very small amount of dehydration," says Amanda Carlson, director of performance nutrition for Athletes' Performance, which trains many of the world's top athletes. "Just losing 2% of your body weight in fluid can decrease performance by up to 25%."[9]

Here are some basic guidelines as suggested by the American Council on Exercise[10] for drinking water before, during, and after exercise:

- Drink 17 to 20 ounces of water 2 to 3 hours before you start exercising.

- Drink 8 ounces of water 20 to 30 minutes before you start exercising.

- Drink 7 to 10 ounces of water every 10 to 20 minutes during exercise.

- Drink 8 ounces of water no more than 30 minutes after you exercise.

WHAT ABOUT SPORTS DRINKS?

If you work out at a high intensity for longer than an hour, you may need more than water to provide nutrients and electrolytes lost during exercise. Choose wisely— they often contain added sugar, sodium, and caffeine. Also check the serving size. One drink can contain 2 or 3 servings, which can double or triple the number of calories and amount of sugar listed on the nutrition label.

Don't wait until you experience the following symptoms of dehydration to take action:

- Dizziness or lightheadedness

- Nausea or vomiting

- Muscle cramps

- Dry mouth

MY JOURNEY

- Lack of sweating

- Hard, fast heartbeat

- Mental confusion

- Weakness

And here are some benefits that come with staying hydrated:

- Water is calorie free, makes you feel full, and helps you eat less, thereby encouraging weight loss.[11]

- Your heart doesn't have to work as hard to pump blood throughout the body.[12]

- Water helps digestion by passing waste through the body, keeping you regular.[13]

- Water flushes toxins from your kidneys.[14]

- Water helps muscle performance.[15]

- Water boosts brain function and mood.[16]

- Water can help and prevent migraines.[17]

Bottom line: Do your body a favor—grab your water bottle and drink up!

GET OUT THERE AND WALK!

Walking is one of the easiest ways to get fit. For most of us, walking comes as naturally as breathing, after all it is one of the first things we learned to do in life—until we wake up and discover that we can't do it like we used to. For some of us, even walking the shortest distance is a challenge.

Regardless of your fitness level, walking is still a great place to start.

- It is inexpensive.
- It can be done anywhere.
- It doesn't require practice or special equipment.

According to a recent study by the U.S. Centers for Disease Control and Prevention, the most popular exercise for individuals wanting to lose weight is walking. Here's how various activities stack up for men and women:

MEN		WOMEN	
Walking	37.7%	Walking	52.5%
Running and Jogging	10.7%	Aerobics	8.7%
Weight lifting	9.6%	Gardening	8.2%
Golfing	8.1%	Exercise machines	8%

Before you get started, let's walk through some easy tips that can reduce your risk of injury and ensure that you get the most out of your workout.
- Stand up straight. Keep your shoulders back and relaxed, chest lifted, and tailbone pointing down to the ground. Look directly ahead. Make sure that your neck and head are centered over your body and not jutting forward.

- Stay relaxed. Relax your shoulders and shake out your arms and wrists. Wiggle your fingers from time to time and swing your arms naturally as you walk. This will help keep any swelling down and your heart rate up.

- Use heel-to-toe motion. As you walk, your heel should be the first part of your foot to hit the ground. Roll through the ball of the foot and push off with your toes. This will reduce the risk of shin splints and tendon pulls.

We recommend two great walking programs to help keep you motivated and to provide a tool for accountability and tracking progress: 10,000 Steps a Day, and the 100-Mile Club.

10,000 STEPS A DAY

Recent studies show the following benefits of 10,000 steps a day:

Walking helps prevent heart disease in women. According to the American Heart Association, heart disease is on the decline in men but on the increase in women. Women are six times more likely to die from heart disease than breast cancer, and heart disease kills more women over age 65 than any other disease.

Walking provides an incentive to increase activity levels. In a recent study, participants who tracked their daily steps tended to walk more every day, even when they were below their goal of 10,000 steps per day.

Walking helps improve overall body composition. Middle-aged women who took at least 10,000 steps per day on average were much more likely to fall into recommended ranges for total body weight and body fat percentage, according to the results of a study published in Medicine and Science in Sports and Exercise. Conversely, inactive women—those taking fewer than 6,000 steps per day—were more likely to be overweight or obese and have a higher waist circumference, which increases the risk of cardiovascular disease.

Working toward 10,000 steps a day is a wonderful way to increase lifestyle activity without having to schedule in exercise time.

MYplace ○ FOR FITNESS

DETERMINE YOUR WALKING CATEGORY

Most sedentary Americans move only about 2,000 to 3,000 steps a day. Studies reveal that increasing the number up to 6,000 steps a day can significantly reduce the risk of death, and 8,000 to 10,000 steps a day promotes weight loss. Wear a fitness tracker or pedometer for a week, and determine which of the following categories describes you:

- Sedentary: 5,000 or fewer steps a day

- Low active: 5,000 to 7,499 steps a day

- Somewhat active: 7,500 to 9,999 steps a day (likely to include some exercise or walking)

- Active or moderately active: 10,000 steps a day

- Highly active: 12,500 or more steps a day

STEP EQUIVALENTS	
1 mile	2,100 average steps
1 block	200 average steps
10 minutes of walking	1,200 steps on average
bicycling or swimming	150 steps per minute
weight lifting	100 steps per minute
roller-skating	200 steps per minute

(source: www.about.com.)

MAKE EVERY STEP COUNT WITH A FITNESS TRACKER

While wearing one isn't essential, keeping track of even small steps can speed you toward your fitness goals. Pedometers are relatively inexpensive fitness tracker. To get the most mileage out of your fitness tracker, keep the following in mind:

- Choose a fitness tracker or pedometer with a display that is easy to read. If you choose to wear a pedometer, choose one that has a clip that stays snugly against your body and won't easily slip or bounce off.

- Establish a baseline of steps by measuring the number of steps you take in an average day. To determine your baseline standard, record your findings for three days, add them up and divide by three.

- Increase your steps gradually (approximately 200 to 1,000 steps a day) by adding to your baseline average.

- Your goal will be 10,000 steps a day, which is approximately 5 miles.

- Shopping can be one way of getting in some steps, but remember that your fitness tracker might be responding to movement as you swing your arms. If you are pushing a cart, you might want to move your tracker to your shoe if possible.

- To ensure that you wear your tracker, keep it in a prominent place, such as your bathroom counter, so that you will remember to snap it on every morning.

THE 100-MILE CLUB

Can't walk that mile yet? Don't be discouraged! Just keep moving! You'll be surprised at how quickly your activity adds up each month. The key is to be consistent. Keep a record of your activity minutes on your Live It Tracker or in your Bible study (the 100-mile chart on the inside back cover). Then convert those minutes to miles, following the chart below. You are not competing with anyone but yourself. Your job is to strive to reach 100 miles before the last meeting in your current First Place for Health group session.

MYplace O FOR FITNESS

WALKING			
slowly, 2 mph	30 min =	156 cal =	1 mile
moderately, 3 mph	20 min =	156 cal =	1 mile
very briskly, 4 mph	15 min =	156 cal =	1 mile
speed walking	10 min =	156 cal =	1 mile
up stairs	13 min =	159 cal =	1 mile
RUNNING / JOGGING			
• • •	10 min =	156 cal =	1 mile
CYCLE OUTDOORS			
slowly, < 10 mph	20 min =	156 cal =	1 mile
light effort, 10-12 mph	12 min =	156 cal =	1 mile
moderate effort, 12-14 mph	10 min =	156 cal =	1 mile
vigorous effort, 14-16 mph	7.5 min =	156 cal =	1 mile
very fast, 16-19 mph	6.5 min =	152 cal =	1 mile
SPORTS ACTIVITIES			
playing tennis (singles)	10 min =	156 cal =	1 mile
swimming			
light to moderate effort	11 min =	152 cal =	1 mile
fast, vigorous effort	7.5 min =	156 cal =	1 mile
softball	15 min =	156 cal =	1 mile
golf	20 min =	156 cal =	1 mile
rollerblading	6.5 min =	152 cal =	1 mile
ice skating	11 min =	152 cal =	1 mile
jumping rope	7.5 min =	156 cal =	1 mile
basketball	12 min =	156 cal =	1 mile
soccer (casual)	15 min =	159 min =	1 mile
AROUND THE HOUSE			
mowing grass	22 min =	156 cal =	1 mile
mopping, sweeping, vacuuming	19.5 min =	155 cal =	1 mile
cooking	40 min =	160 cal =	1 mile
gardening	19 min =	156 cal =	1 mile
housework (general)	35 min =	156 cal =	1 mile

AROUND THE HOUSE			
ironing	45 min =	153 cal =	1 mile
raking leaves	25 min =	150 cal =	1 mile
washing car	23 min =	156 cal =	1 mile
washing dishes	45 min =	153 cal =	1 mile
AT THE GYM			
stair machine	8.5 min =	155 cal =	1 mile
stationary bike			
slowly, 10 mph	30 min =	156 cal =	1 mile
moderately, 10-13 mph	15 min =	156 cal =	1 mile
vigorously, 13-16 mph	7.5 min =	156 cal =	1 mile
briskly, 16-19 mph	6.5 min =	156 cal =	1 mile
elliptical trainer	12 min =	156 cal =	1 mile
weight machines (vigorously)	13 min =	152 cal =	1 mile
aerobics			
low impact	15 min =	156 cal =	1 mile
high impact	12 min =	156 cal =	1 mile
water	20 min =	156 cal =	1 mile
pilates	15 min =	156 cal =	1 mile
raquetball (casual)	15 min =	156 cal =	1 mile
stretching exercises	25 min =	150 cal =	1 mile
weight lifting (also works for weight machines used moderately or gently)	30 min =	156 cal =	1 mile
FAMILY LEISURE			
playing piano	37 min =	155 cal =	1 mile
jumping rope	10 min =	152 cal =	1 mile
skating (moderate)	20 min =	152 cal =	1 mile
swimming			
moderate	17 min =	156 cal =	1 mile
vigorous	10 min =	148 cal =	1 mile
table tennis	25 min =	150 cal =	1 mile
walk / run / play with kids	25 min =	150 cal =	1 mile

MYplace O FOR FITNESS

GET STARTED WITH A WALKING PROGRAM

Getting started with either of the walking programs—10,000 Steps a Day or the 100-Mile Club—is easy, and there are only a few basic things that you'll need:

- A good pair of walking shoes—Walking shoes do not have to be expensive, but they do need to have a lot of stability and plenty of space in the toe box for wiggle room.

- Appropriate undergarments—A pair of lycra bike shorts helps prevent chaffing, and a good sports bra offers the support you need. Chaffing powders and lotions can be purchased at any sporting-goods store.

- Fitness tracker—A fitness tracker is optional, but it offers accountability and helps you see the progress you are making. Numbers don't lie.

- Positive attitude—A positive attitude in not an option. It is mandatory!

To maximize your walking program, consider the following suggestions:

- When taking a walk, go to the end of the sidewalk and all the way around the cul-de-sac—no shortcuts!

- Walk while you talk on the phone. Keep a steady pace.

- Use small chunks of time. If you only have 10 minutes, get out there and do it! Three 10-minute walks have the same health benefits as one 30-minute walk.

- Keep an extra pair of walking shoes in the car. Take advantage of situations when you are stuck somewhere.

- Get out of the car. Don't wait in the car when you are picking up your kids from practice. Arrive early and walk.

- Make your walk an extension of your quiet time. After completing your Bible study, head out the door for your prayer time. It's the best type of multi-tasking there is.

MY JOURNEY

To find out how many calories you burn walking:

1. Find your weight on the left

2. Find the speed you walk on the right

The corresponding number is the number of calories burned per hour.

WEIGHT (IN LBS.)	MILES PER HOUR				
	2	2.5	3	4	4.5
100	114	136	159	182	205
105	119	143	167	191	215
100	114	136	159	182	205
105	119	143	167	191	215
110	125	150	175	200	225
115	131	157	183	209	235
120	136	164	191	218	245
125	142	170	199	227	256
130	148	177	207	236	266
135	153	184	215	245	276
140	159	191	223	255	286
145	165	198	231	264	297
150	170	205	239	273	307
155	176	211	247	282	317
160	182	218	255	291	327
165	188	225	263	300	338
170	193	232	270	309	348

MYplace O FOR FITNESS

WEIGHT (IN LBS.)	MILES PER HOUR				
	2	2.5	3	4	4.5
180	205	245	286	327	368
185	210	252	294	336	378
190	216	259	302	345	389
200	227	273	318	364	409
205	233	280	326	373	419
210	239	286	334	382	430
215	244	293	342	391	440
220	250	300	350	400	450
225	256	307	358	409	460
230	261	314	366	418	470
235	267	320	374	427	481
240	273	327	382	436	491
245	278	334	390	445	501
250	284	341	398	455	511
255	290	348	406	464	522
260	295	355	414	473	532
265	301	361	422	482	542
270	307	368	430	491	552
275	313	375	438	500	563
280	318	382	445	509	573
285	324	389	453	518	583
290	330	395	461	527	593
295	335	402	469	536	603
300	341	409	477	545	614

FIT YOUR FEET—10 TIPS FOR CHOOSING THE RIGHT ATHLETIC SHOE FOR YOU

Does it ever seem like you need an advanced degree to know which shoe to buy for a workout? You drive to the sporting-goods store and stand there looking at the countless numbers of cross-trainers, running shoes, walking shoes, court shoes, hiking shoes—it seems to go on and on. Then there are neutral, stability, and motion control—what's that about? Choosing the right shoe for the right activity is key to keeping your feet happy. Conversely, not choosing the right shoe for your feet could leave you with shin splints or painful heels that cause you to abandon your workout routine. Here are 13 tips to help you choose just the right shoe and keep you on track.[18]

1. **Don't make shoes multitask.** A walking shoe is stiffer than a running shoe. A tennis shoe has a smooth shoe bottom to allow ease of movement. If you plan on doing different activities, get a pair that is right for that activity.

2. **Measure your foot frequently.** "It's a myth that foot size doesn't change in adults," says Steven Raiken, MD. "It does change as we get older, so have your feet measured twice a year. Sizes also vary between brands, so go by what fits, not by what size the shoe is." (Raiken is director of the foot and ankle service at the Rothman Institute at Thomas Jefferson University Hospital in Philadelphia.)

3. **Shop late in the day when your feet are their largest** (feet swell during the day).

4. **Bring your own socks and orthotics.** Using the socks provided in a store may not reflect the thickness of the socks you normally wear. Orthotics will affect the thickness within the shoe. Always remove the insert that comes with the shoe when placing your orthotic into the shoe.

5. **Shop according to your foot.** Feet come in all shapes, sizes and widths. Some have high arches; others don't. Your feet deserve to be comfortable. After all, they'll be doing some hard work. Most major brands offer various models to fit all foot types.

WET FOOTPRINT TEST
FOOT ARCH TYPES

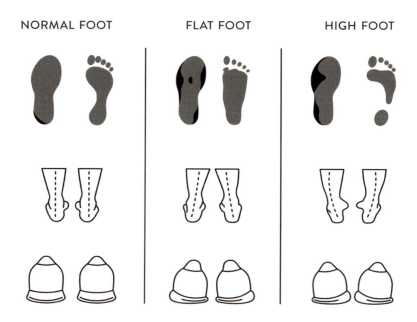

The "wet test" will help you determine your foot shape. To perform the wet test, use a large piece of brown paper, such as a large grocery sack. Wet your foot and quickly step onto the paper, leaving your footprint. Trace the wet footprint. This will reveal whether you have high arches, a neutral foot, or low arches. High arches will leave a footprint that has a minimal connection between the forefoot and heel. This means you under-pronate (roll your foot to the outside), which will cause wear on the outside edge of your shoe and heel. A neutral foot will have a distinct curve and your shoes will wear evenly. Low arches (or flat feet) will have a large footprint with little or no curve, so your shoes might wear more on the inside edge.

6. **Measure your foot while standing, and make sure you have enough room in the toe box to curl your toes up without discomfort.** Your toes should not rub up against the front of the shoe. The rule of thumb is a half-inch of space between your toe and the end of the shoe. The American Academy of Orthopedic Surgeons recommends that when fitting into an athletic shoe you should be able to freely wiggle all of your toes when the shoe is on.

7. **Measure both of your feet.** Most people have one foot that is slightly larger than the other. Fit your shoe to the larger foot.

8. **Always choose comfort** over how cute the shoe is or how the shoe makes your foot look. If they hurt in the store, don't buy them, no matter how trendy they are. With so many styles on the market, you are sure to find one that is fashionable as well as the perfect fit for your foot.

9. **Don't be afraid to break them in.** Try them out in the store. Walk around, or take a jog down the aisle. Ask yourself how they feel and where they hit your arch. Make sure they feel good in motion. As a fitness instructor, you'll often find me doing a variety of moves when trying on new shoes.

10. **If you are working out three times a week, you need to replace your shoes approximately every 500 miles or every 6 months.** Wear your athletic shoes only for working out. They will last much longer if you don't wear them for everyday activities. Grab a sharpie and write the date you purchased your shoes on the tongue of the new shoe. It's a great way to keep track of their age and know when to replace them.

11. **Buy your next pair of shoes before your old pair wears out.** Or buy two pairs of shoes if you find a style that really works for you. Styles are discontinued quickly.

12. **Exercising in worn-out shoes can contribute to injuries.** A new pair of shoes is a lot cheaper than knee surgery.

13. **Over-the-counter orthotics can be a great option if you find you need additional arch support.** Find a store that will allow you to try different-sized orthotics. Stand on several different sizes of orthotics to find the one that fits your foot. The length can be cut to fit your shoe but you can't change where the arch hits. Find the one that fits you. My shoe size is a 9 but my orthotic has been a 10 and sometimes an 11, depending on the brand.

Here is a little bit more information (taken from *Podiatry Today*):

Running shoes. These shoes are lightest in weight and offer maximum cushioning. They are designed for linear activity and should never be worn for court activity. Running shoes are acceptable for walking but walking shoes are never acceptable for running.

Walking shoes. Similar to running shoes, athletic walking shoes often have more leather in the upper, making them more durable and slightly heavier. These shoes generally are not as boldly designed and are often more appropriate for everyday wear.

Court shoes. Tennis, basketball and other court sports require quick changes in direction. Accordingly, these shoes must have superior medial and lateral forefoot support. Tennis also entails a lot of forefoot dragging, so this type of court shoe often features extra thickness in the big-toe area.

Cross-training shoes. These versatile shoes generally come in two different versions: lighter-weight models similar to running shoes and those similar to court shoes. Lightweight cross-trainers are OK for running up to three miles and for use on exercise machines. For basketball, tennis and other court activities, the heavier-weight cross-trainer, often made from leather, is better.

Hiking shoes. Hiking requires support, durability and protection from the environment. Such shoes feature thicker soles and come up higher on the foot to increase ankle support. Waterproof lining and sealed seams keep the feet dry.[19]

LACING YOUR SHOES FOR COMFORT

You've purchased the perfect shoe. We've all been taught how to tie our shoelaces, but what about lacing them for the most comfort? Making a few simple adjustments in how you lace your shoes for your foot type and arch can prevent foot fatigue and nagging pain, and can provide stability and support. Because I have a wide forefoot, I have found that lacing my shoe accordingly has significantly decreased pain at the widest part of my foot. Take a look at the diagram below and try a new lacing technique to fit your foot type and see if you find similar results.

BORN TO RUN?

In the 1970s, Bruce Springsteen sang "Baby, you were born to run." And we all did—as children. We ran in the streets, playgrounds and parks, never thinking a thing about how hard it was—because it was a natural part of playing. But as we grew, running and playing began to change. We started to walk more, run less, play organized sports, or not play sports at all. Now as adults we wonder if we might ever have the desire to run again. What was once so natural as a kid now seems like a chore.

I would often see people jogging/running on the side of the road and wish that I could do the same. Some seemed to move effortlessly, like they were gliding along. It looked like they could run forever. If you, like me, want to run, I'm here to tell you that you can. There is hope. I started with walk/run intervals. I would walk for 2 or 3 minutes and run for 30 seconds. I started with a mile. Over time, I was able to reduce the walk intervals to 1 minute and increase the run intervals to 1 minute. This was a comfortable pace for me, so that's where I stayed. I eventually increased my running distance to 3 miles.

Running can be a great form of exercise.

- It can be done almost anywhere and anytime.
- It takes little skill.
- It needs a good pair of shoes.
- It burns a higher number of calories in a shorter amount of time.
- It can be done alone, with a partner, or in a group.
- It's a good option if you are ready to increase your workout.

Today, running has become a popular choice for people. There are running clubs and groups you can join, apps that will take you from the couch to a 5K, and triathlons for those who want to combine it with biking and swimming. You can run for a cause or just run for enjoyment. But whatever your fitness level or reason for running, the opportunities are endless.

MYplace ○ FOR FITNESS

LACING YOUR SHOES FOR COMFORT

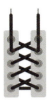

HEEL SLIPPING
RESULT: Ankle gets more support with comfortable fit.

WIDE FOREFOOT
RESULT: The forefoot gets more space in the toe box.

WIDE FEET IN GENERAL
RESULT: Loosens the shoe and gives the foot more space.

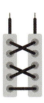

NARROW FOOT
RESULT: Tightens the shoe more than the traditional tying technique.

SHOES FEEL TOO TIGHT
RESULT: The laces will be evenly distributed for a more comfortable fit.

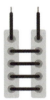

TOE PAIN & BLACK TOE NAILS
RESULT: The toe box will be lifted giving the toes more space.

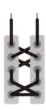

HIGH ARCHES HIGH MIDFOOT
RESULT: The middle section will minimize pressure and add comfort to the fit.

As with any activity, there are some things to remember when you start out:

1. **Start safely.** Talk with your doctor before beginning. He/she will help you determine what activity best fits your health and fitness level.

2. **Invest in a good pair of running shoes.** (See the "Fit Your Feet" section about buying proper athletic shoes.) Before you need other accessories, such as a GPS watch, fitness tracker, or specialized apparel, you need a good pair of running shoes. They are the best investment you can make for your feet. There are specialty stores that will help you find the perfect shoe for your stride and foot.

3. **Start slowly and set realistic expectations.** Most running injuries are caused by doing too much too soon. If you've been sedentary or are new to running, start by walking. As your fitness level increases, add in a few jogging intervals. Walk to a mailbox or stop sign, and then jog to the next one. Or walk for one minute, and then run/jog for 30 seconds. Repeat 10 times or so. Do this twice a week at first to see how you do and increase as you are able. Don't expect that you'll be ready for a 5K in a week or so. Set small, winnable goals.

4. **Remember the three Cs of running: comfortable, controlled and conversational.** Running is almost always steady-state exercise, meaning you maintain a fairly constant pace. You should be able to carry on a conversation when running with a partner. If you can't, and you find yourself panting for air, then you need to slow down and control your pace to a more comfortable one.

5. **Do dynamic movement instead of static stretching.** Traditionally, static stretching (holding a muscle in a stretched, fixed position for about 30 seconds) has been used to warm up your muscles before a run. Jason Fitzgerald, USATF-certified running coach and founder of Strength Running, says that an easy three-to-five-minute dynamic warm-up will "prepare you by lubricating joints, increasing heart rate, warming muscles, opening capillaries, and getting the central nervous system primed for running." This type of warm-up has been shown to reduce your risk of injury. (See the section on stretching and warm-up.) Static stretching can be used after your workout is complete. Concentrate on stretches that focus on legs, ankles, calves, core, back and hips.

6. **Stay relaxed when you run.** Keep your back straight, shoulders back, and head up. Swing your arms freely at about the level of your hips, and keep

MYplace ⭘ **FOR FITNESS**

your hands relaxed. Breathe through your nose or mouth naturally, focusing on diaphragmatic (core) breathing, instead of shallow breaths or chest breathing. Land on your heel, keep your toes pointed forward, roll your foot forward, and push off with the ball of your foot. Maintain a smooth stride and avoid bouncing.

7. **Stay hydrated!** Drink plenty of water before, during and after your run. Don't wait until you feel thirsty to drink.

8. **Listen to your body.** If anything hurts, take time off or slow your pace until it feels better. Plan rest days to allow your body to recover and to minimize overuse injuries.

9. **Stay motivated with music.** Load up your phone or MP3 player with energetic music that will keep you moving to the beat. Music can be highly motivating, especially when you listen to your favorites. If you are taking it outdoors, make sure it's not so loud that you can't hear an approaching car or another runner.

10. **Use an app to track your progress.** An app such as Map My Run will track your distance and time, and will allow you to include notes about how you felt during your workout, or anything else that might be helpful as you look back and see how far you've come.

11. **Vary your workouts on your days off.** Add in some strength-training, body-weight exercises, or core training to reduce your risk of injury and to increase your strength so that running is easier and more comfortable. (See "Strength Training 101" section.)

12. **Choose the right clothing.** Chances are good that if you make running a part of your exercise routine, you'll battle the elements at some point.

   — In hot weather: Clothing should be lightweight and loose-fitting. Light-colored clothing is usually best. The new fabrics that wick away moisture won't add additional heaviness from sweat like cotton can. Sunglasses, a cap and sunscreen are important.

   — In colder weather: Wear several lightweight layers rather than one heavy layer. The inner layer should be a fabric that wicks moisture away from your body. Choose an outer layer that blocks the wind and moisture. As your body warms up, you can remove a layer of clothing. Don't forget your hat and gloves. Large amounts of body heat are lost through an exposed head.

MY JOURNEY

— Make yourself visible: If running at dusk or nighttime, always wear bright, reflective clothing. Headlamps are a popular accessory and will allow you to see comfortably in front of you and offer more noticeability to any traffic.

13. **You can run anywhere**—in your neighborhood, at the park, on a track or treadmill. Wherever you choose to run, be sure it's convenient, enjoyable and safe. Consider the following when choosing a location:

— Choose a place with little traffic and few obstacles.

— Always try to run against traffic so that you can see approaching vehicles.

— At night, run on well-lit streets in a familiar neighborhood, and consider taking a partner with you.

— Always let someone know where you are going and when you will return.

— Make sure to wear light-colored and reflective clothing, and add a headlamp.

— A track can be a great place to run. It has a special surface, you're never too far from where you started, and you can easily measure your distance. On a regular-sized track, four laps will equal a mile.

— It's best to run on smooth and flat surfaces to lower your risk of injury.

A Sample Program

Here are a few quick reminders as you begin your new program:

○ If you are an absolute beginner to running, start by walking briskly for at least 20 to 30 minutes several days a week before moving on to a running program.

○ When you're ready to begin, consider running short distances during your walk.

○ Try to work out at least three days each week of the program.

○ If you find a particular week's pattern tiring, repeat it before going on to the next level.

○ Progress according to your goals and how you feel. There is no rush to complete the program in 12 weeks.

MYplace O FOR FITNESS

WEEK	WARM UP (RIDE SLOWLY)	AEROBIC CYCLING (RIDE MODERATELY TO VIGOROUSLY)	COOL DOWN (RIDE SLOWLY)	TOTAL TIME
1	5 minutes	5 minutes 1 minute	5 minutes	20-30 minutes
2	5 minutes	5 minutes 1 minute	5 minutes	20-30 minutes
3	5 minutes	5 minutes 2 minutes	5 minutes	25 minutes
4	5 minutes	4 minutes 2 minutes	5 minutes	20-30 minutes
5	5 minutes	5 minutes 3 minutes	5 minutes	20-30 minutes
6	5 minutes	4 minutes 3 minutes	5 minutes	20-30 minutes
7	5 minutes	5 minutes 5 minutes	5 minutes	20-30 minutes
8	5 minutes	5 minutes 8 minutes	5 minutes	20-30 minutes
9	5 minutes	10 minutes 10 minutes	5 minutes	30 minutes
10	5 minutes	5 minutes 15 minutes	5 minutes	30 minutes
11	5 minutes	20 minutes	5 minutes	30 minutes

MY JOURNEY

WEEK 12

Congratulations! You've reached the 12-week point and are running 20 minutes three days per week. You might feel like you are ready for more. If so, add another day of walking or jogging. Start with week 1 and follow the schedule for increasing your time on that day. If not, stay where you are. At this pace, you are achieving the aerobic benefits you need for good health.

Other tips to remember:

- Increase your pace gradually over a period of several weeks. One way to increase your pace is to use interval training. Run faster for one to three minutes and then slow down for three to five minutes or until your breathing has returned to normal. Start with one interval each workout; then add an interval each week, or when you're ready.

- Increase your running time by three to five minutes each week or as you feel ready.

- Consider cross-training with another activity, such as swimming, bicycling, HIIT, or strength training.

- Remember, running isn't for everyone. Don't give up on exercise if running isn't something you enjoy. There are lots of other workouts to consider. Try something else. But just keep moving!

I don't *love* running, but I don't hate it either, and I am always proud of the workout I accomplished when I'm done.

MYplace ○ FOR FITNESS

BICYCLING YOUR WAY TO HEALTH AND FITNESS

There's an old adage, "It's like riding a bike." This is often used to explain muscle memory—how a learned activity becomes something you never forget how to do.

How long has it been since you've pedaled a bicycle? Do you remember as a kid the day the training wheels came off? You struggled to control the handlebars and stay upright. But before long you were pedaling down the road as fast as you could, pulling your feet away from the pedals and gliding down the street with the wind in your hair.

The sport of cycling has advanced tremendously over the last few decades. Today, you can compete in a myriad of triathlons or cycling competitions if you want to, or you can simply enjoy a leisurely ride with a friend or loved one. The benefits are the same and you don't have to be Lance Armstrong to enjoy them!

- It is low impact—easy on the bones and joints.

- It strengthens the muscles of the lower body, such as the quadriceps, hamstrings, hips, gluteals, and calves.

- It engages the core constantly.

- The upper body and arms get a workout when climbing hills or riding a stationary bike with arm levers.

- It can give you a wonderful sense of accomplishment; it gives you time away from the busyness of life; and it gets you in touch with nature, especially when you are outdoors.

- It's versatile. It can be done indoors or outdoors.

Before purchasing a bike, ask yourself the following questions:

- Do I want to ride indoors or outdoors?

- Do I plan to ride long distances—greater than 20 miles?

MY JOURNEY

- Will I be competing in cycling events?

- Will I be riding in the neighborhood, on a bike trail (paved or dirt), or on country roads?

- How much money do I want to spend? Bicycles can range from $150 to more than $2,000. Once you purchase your bike, check it each time before you ride to ensure that it's in good repair.

Outdoor Bicycles

- Racing bicycles are lightweight and have narrow tires and dropped handlebars. Most have 10 to 14 gears.

- Mountain bicycles are very popular because they can be used on or off road. They have wide tires and upright handlebars, and they provide a softer ride than racing bikes. They have from 18 to 24 gears.

- Hybrid bicycles are a cross between a racing and a mountain bike.

- Unless you plan to ride only short distances on flat roads, buy a bicycle with 10 or more gears.

Stationary Bicycles

- Stationary bicycles are relatively inexpensive and can fit in almost any room in the house, and they provide a great way of working out when the weather is bad or your time is limited.

- Choose a bike with a smooth pedaling motion.

- Make sure that you're comfortable with the pedaling resistance and that it's easily adjusted.

- A comfortable and adjustable (tilt) seat is a must. A recumbent bike will provide lower back support.

- Some bikes have arm levers that allow you to work your upper body, too.

MYplace ○ FOR FITNESS

The Proper Fit

○ You are more likely to stick with your exercise program and avoid injuries if you have a bicycle that fits. A specialty shop can help you select a bike that meets your needs.

○ The handlebars should be in a position that allows you to relax your shoulders and arms. You should be able to reach the brake levers easily.

○ Position your feet so that the balls of your feet are in the center of the pedals. If your seat is too high, your hips will rock back and forth when you pedal. A seat that's too low puts extra stress on your knees.

○ The tilt of the saddle should be parallel to the ground. If the seat is tilted downward, you'll have to use your arms to hold your body up. A seat that's tilted too high puts too much pressure on your crotch.

Riding Gear

While not necessary, special cycling clothing can make your ride more fun and have you looking like you belong in the Tour de France.

○ Bicycling shorts are a good investment no matter what type of riding you plan to do. You can buy tight or loose-fitting shorts with a special pad that provides cushioning, absorbs moisture, and prevents chafing.

○ Bicycling shirts are good for riding outdoors because they're tight fitting and cut down on wind resistance. The newer fabrics wick away moisture from your body. Bike shirts may also have special pockets for a water bottle.

○ Bicycling gloves improve comfort by providing padding for your hands.

○ Shoes can really make a difference. Tennis shoes will do the trick, but cycling shoes are lightweight and can improve the efficiency of your pedaling. If you plan to ride longer distances, these are a must. Some cycling pedals and shoes are designed to work together. These take more skill to use because the shoes actually clip directly into the pedals; this provides consistent and more efficient use of energy throughout the pedaling cycle. Never cycle barefoot.

MY JOURNEY

- Sunglasses or protective eyewear for the weather conditions or bugs and insects is important. Even if the sun is not shining brightly, UV rays can be damaging to unprotected eyes, and the last thing you want is a bug in your eye as you are cruising down the road.

- Carry along one or two water bottles. You need to drink water frequently when bicycling. Because of the airflow, you may not realize you're sweating.

Selecting a Helmet

A helmet is your most important piece of equipment. Helmets save lives. Never ride without one!

- Your helmet should fit snugly and comfortably.

- It should have adjustable straps that can be buckled below your jaw.

- The helmet must be certified by the American National Standards Institute (ANSI) or the Snell Foundation.

Other safety considerations include avoiding riding in high-traffic areas or at night and keeping your bike in good repair.

A Sample Bicycling Program

Try to ride at least three days during each week of the program. You don't have to complete the cycling program in eight weeks. If you don't feel ready to move to the next week, then don't. Progress according to your goals and how you feel, but always keep challenging yourself. A brisk ride increases your breathing slightly but not so much that you can't carry on a conversation.

MYplace O FOR FITNESS

WEEK	WARM UP (RIDE SLOWLY)	AEROBIC CYCLING (RIDE MODERATELY TO VIGOROUSLY)	COOL DOWN (RIDE SLOWLY)	TOTAL TIME
1	5 minutes	10 minutes	5 minutes	20 minutes
2	5 minutes	12 minutes	5 minutes	22 minutes
3	5 minutes	15 minutes	5 minutes	25 minutes
4	5 minutes	17 minutes	5 minutes	27 minutes
5	5 minutes	20 minutes	5 minutes	30 minutes
6	5 minutes	25 minutes	5 minutes	35 minutes
7	5 minutes	30 minutes	5 minutes	40 minutes

Once you get to 30 minutes of brisk cycling, you may want to consider some new options:

o Increase the number of days you ride. Ride 4 days instead of 3, or 5 days instead of 4. Ride 4 days one week and then 5 days the following week. Vary your routine.

o A fun option is to do interval training. Ride faster for one to three minutes; then slow down for three to five minutes or until your breathing has returned to normal. Start with one interval each workout, then add an interval each week or when you're ready. Use a timer and sprint for 45 seconds; then slow down for 15 seconds. Repeat this for four rounds and you will have done a Tabata interval. (This is a great workout on a stationary bike.)

o Increase the time you spend riding by three to five minutes each week as you feel ready.

"THE
ONLY BAD
WORKOUT
IS THE ONE
YOU DIDN'T DO"

MYplace ○ FOR FITNESS

5 REASONS YOU AREN'T LOSING WEIGHT: PLATEAUS, STALLS AND ALL-OUT STANDSTILLS—HOW TO BREAK THROUGH

You're working hard—tracking and counting calories and portion sizes, and exercising. Then it all stops—the scale seems to stand still. Sound familiar? There is nothing worse than giving it all you've got and not seeing results.

The truth is that everyone hits plateaus. You are not alone. And while getting past them can be challenging, it's not impossible. Let's look at what could be causing them and how to overcome and get things moving again in the right direction.

You aren't including strength/resistance training. During weight loss, your body loses fat and muscle. Strength training keeps you from losing muscle (actually adds muscle) and gives you the added benefit of increasing your metabolism, which keeps you burning fat long after your workout is done. Don't skip this. Many women believe that if they strength train, they will bulk up like men. While it's true women will develop muscle definition, they simply do not have the testosterone needed to bulk up.[20]

You're doing the same old exercise routine. Chances are, if you are doing the same exercise routine each day, your muscles may have become more efficient, which means they don't need to work as hard. Add some variety and mix things up a bit. Try a different type of workout, such as HIIT, which keeps your muscles strong while burning fat at the same time. Or maybe you need to increase the amount of weight you use when strength training and get those muscles working hard again.[21]

Your metabolism has slowed down. Your smaller self requires less energy expenditure. This can result in a slower metabolism. The same number of calories you needed to lose weight may now just maintain your weight. Try increasing the number of days or minutes you spend exercising. Even one day might be the answer to your breakthrough.

You aren't getting enough sleep. Lack of sleep can result in lack of muscle recovery time and increased stress. When you're tired, you may not want to exercise. "Sleep is an essential ingredient of a healthy lifestyle," says Phyllis Zee, a professor of neurology, neurobiology, and physiology at Northwestern's Feinberg School of Medicine. "Sleep is a barometer of health, like someone's temperature." Zee says that "exercise is good for metabolism, weight management, cardiovascular health, and good for sleep."[22] Do your body a favor and strive for 7-8 hours of sleep a night. Your health is more important than whatever is distracting you from getting that.

You aren't tracking your food accurately or your portion sizes have increased. Plateaus provide a great opportunity to reassess where you are. Are you tracking everything you eat? Are you allowing your portion sizes to creep up? Are you tracking all those hidden calories, such as cream in your coffee or one teaspoon of oil in the pan? Looking at your overall health and wellness plan and making a few adjustments can get you started again.

MYplace ○ FOR FITNESS

MAKING A SPLASH

Bored with your current fitness routine? Jump in and make a splash. Take your workout from the gym to the pool and experience the endless benefits of water workouts. From swimming laps to aqua aerobics to deep-water jogging to interval swimming, there are so many possibilities today.

And while it might not be the first workout you think of when it comes to weight loss, with its calorie burn, boost in metabolism, and muscle recruitment, it should be. Water workouts can be done almost every day without risk of injury because this type of exercise is so gentle on your body. Without putting stress on the joints, water workouts build lean muscle, increase cardiovascular capacity, and offer a resistance workout for one's core, hips, glutes, arms and shoulders.

But let's face it, if you're struggling with weight, the thought of a pool can be frightening. Getting into a swimsuit probably isn't on your top 10 lists of things to do. Don't let this stop you! Today there are so many alternatives to the swimsuits of old. You have swim shorts, swim skirts, tankinis, and swim dresses, just to name a few. And guys and gals alike can enjoy rash guards and sun shirts that are specifically made for the water and provide much-needed cover. And if the thought of getting your hair wet makes you a little anxious, you'll be glad to know that swim caps are back in style.

Most health clubs, YMCAs and community centers also offer a variety of aqua fit classes. These classes are designed for all age groups and abilities and are easy on the joints. It's also a great choice for pregnant women, people who easily overheat, and those who need a safe way to be active.

Water workouts use the same basic movements as regular aerobics classes. And, in addition to being a beneficial physical activity, this is a great way to enjoy the friendship that comes from working out with a group.

Water is great for exercise because it:

○ provides resistance

○ keeps you cool (you won't even know you're sweating)

○ supports your body weight

Did you know that if you stand with the water at waist height, your body bears about 50 percent of its body weight? Take the water level to your chest and it will bear about 25 percent of your body weight, and at neck level about 10 percent. This buoyancy allows you to truly customize your workout for your needs.

Getting in the water can offer some incredible benefits:

- decreases body fat

- improves body awareness, balance and coordination

- increases flexibility and muscle strength

- improves cardiovascular fitness

- is low impact and has a lower risk of injury

- improves mood and self-esteem

- is fun and enjoyable

Different Types of Water Exercise

Water Aerobics—Water aerobics classes often feature vertical exercises that mimic land exercises, such as walking, running and even kickboxing.

Deep-water Exercise—This is done in the deep end of the pool and involves running, jogging, and more, using a flotation device. This type of water exercise makes an excellent HIIT workout.

Lap Swimming—Just what it says it is, but you can turn this into a HIIT routine by varying the speed from lap to lap. Or you can add variety by changing up the type of stroke with each lap.

Resistance Training Workouts—Think yoga, Pilates, or tai chi in a pool. This type of workout incorporates these kinds of movements.

Sport-specific Workouts—Are you conditioning for a specific sport? Water workouts allow you to target certain parts of your body while adding variety to your normal routine.

MYplace **O** FOR FITNESS

Prescriptive Workouts—Good News! Doctors have been prescribing this for years. If you battle fibromyalgia, arthritis, osteoporosis, back pain or joint pain, these conditions don't have to keep you down. In fact, several studies have shown that exercising in water offers reduced pain, improved functionality, and better emotional health.

Here are some ideas to help get you going if you want to go it alone:

- Simply start at one end of the pool and walk back and forth from end to end.

- Increase the intensity by swinging your arms back and forth in the water.

- Take it deeper—the deeper the water, the greater the resistance and the more you rely on your balance.

- Buy a flotation vest for deep-water running. Water gloves, water weights and similar equipment can be used to add variety to your workout.

- Rest between laps; keep it an active rest by walking.

- As you become fitter, you can increase the speed and distance you swim.

- Work up to about 30 minutes of moderate to vigorous movement in the water.

- Use a modified breaststroke or backstroke that allows you to keep your head out of the water and a frog-like kick for mobility.

- Once coordination and fitness improve, add a freestyle (front crawl) stroke.

- It's all about comfort. Goggles, earplugs, caps, snorkels and fins may make you feel more relaxed in the water.

- Stay hydrated. Even though you're surrounded by water, don't forget to drink. Keep a water bottle nearby so that you can hydrate while you exercise.

MY JOURNEY

Try this HIIT lap-swim workout:

1. Swim 100 meters using any stroke you like. This is your warm-up. Your goal is to gradually increase your speed as you move through the workout. Enjoy the leisurely pace during this phase.

2. Rest 30 seconds.

3. Swim another 100 meters. Let your focus be on your core. Be intentional with every movement.

4. Rest 30 seconds.

5. Here's where you start to move into intervals. Swim 100 meters 5 times resting 30 seconds in between each set. For the first 50 meters, swim at a good pace, and then increase your pace for the next 50 meters.

6. Swim another 100 meters using the freestyle stroke again. This time make it a competition with yourself and try to beat this time in future swim HIIT sessions. Go for it! Swim hard.

7. Rest 30 seconds.

8. Swim 50 meters. (5x) Swim with any stroke, focusing on kicking to gain speed with each set. Rest 30 seconds after each set.

9. Swim 100 meters, or more if needed, to cool down. Use any stroke you enjoy.

Well done! You've just completed your first HIIT water workout!

TAKING IT OUTSIDE!

One of the best parts of exercising outdoors is just being outside. Running, hiking, biking, skiing, kayaking, tennis—the list can go on and on. There's something about the fresh air and being outside that makes a workout just a bit more invigorating.

But being outside also exposes you to things that you won't find in a nice comfy, air-conditioned gym. Here are a few precautions to take when taking your workout outside.

Plan your water. How long will you be outside and what type of exercise will you be doing? Short workouts just need water, but if you are training for a marathon or playing a sport, you may need to include some electrolytes. (See "Water: The Everyday Guzzle" for guidance on staying hydrated.)

Protect your head. Biking? Make sure you wear a helmet. But what about other activities? Don't let your head go uncovered and risk unwanted sun exposure. Wear a well-ventilated baseball cap or other type of hat to protect yourself from harmful UV rays.

Use sunscreen. Make sure you apply it 30 minutes before your workout, and don't forget to rub it onto the tops of your ears as well.

Check the air-quality standards if you live in a city where pollution runs high. Consider taking your workout inside on days when levels are over 100.

If you are used to working out inside, you may want to lighten your workout on hotter days. Give your body time to adjust to the outside temperatures. It takes 10-14 days for your body to adjust. Or work out first thing in the morning or after the sun starts to set. In any case, if you feel yourself getting dizzy, drink water and get out of the heat.

Choose the right shoes. What activity do you plan on doing? Hiking boots are, well, great for hiking. They offer support around the ankle and lateral movements. But they aren't so good for tennis. So, choose the appropriate shoe for the exercise. Refer to the section titled "Fit Your Feet." All the same principles apply.

MY JOURNEY

Layer your clothing. Not only do weather conditions change but so too does your body temperature. Wear clothing that can be easily removed or put back on, and make sure each layer has reflective accents so that you can easily be seen.

Wear a headlamp or carry a flashlight. Headlamps are lightweight and easy to wear, freeing up your hands. But a good old-fashioned flashlight will also do the trick.

Consider how you are going to carry necessities. A lot of athletic clothes have pockets to store keys and credit cards or a small amount of money. If yours don't, consider carrying a small backpack or fanny pack to store these things or even some extra clothing.

When exercising in the heat, avoid clothing that doesn't ventilate well, such as rubberized suits or sweat suits. You laugh, but people do it. It's a dangerous practice that can lead to dehydration and heatstroke!

Don't rely only on the thermometer! Windchill greatly increases the chill your body experiences. Activities such as roller-blading, ice skating, skiing and even running can contribute to a heightened windchill factor.

Wear an outer layer that keeps out the wind and moisture. Wool and synthetic fabrics are good choices for working out in the cold because they wick moisture away from your body.

Dress appropriately for cold and inclement weather. During the colder months, much of your body's heat can be lost through your head and neck, so wear a hat and scarf. Don't forget to protect your hands.

Watch out for slick surfaces caused by rain and snow.

Be safe. When exercising in the cold, stay close to home or other shelter and always let someone know where you are going.

HOT-WEATHER ALERT

Take precautions when the humidity is above 70 percent and the temperature is above 70 degrees. According to the American Heart Association, weather conditions can be hard on your heart. When you sweat, you lose fluid. Your heart has

MYplace O FOR FITNESS

to pump even harder to get a smaller volume of blood to your working muscles, skin and other body parts. Extreme fluid loss can lead to brain and heart damage.

Check your body-fluid level the morning *after* exercising outdoors. If you weigh two pounds less than usual, you may be dehydrated and need to drink more water—especially if you plan to engage in more outdoor activity!

A Note About Altitude

Altitude increases the stress of physical activity. It's harder for your body to take in oxygen above 5,000 feet. This means that your heart, lungs and muscles have to work harder. Symptoms of altitude sickness include lightheadedness, dizziness, nausea, and unusual shortness of breath. Give yourself a couple of days to get used to the higher elevation, and cut back the intensity of your activities.

HOW TO LOOK CHIC DURING YOUR WORKOUT

Wear clothes that flatter your figure. Gone are the days when, if you were overweight, your only option was a baggy T-shirt. Today, anyone can be fashionable with active wear that you can be comfortable in too. In fact, experts say that putting on a flattering outfit motivates people to exercise in public.

And while just about every store offers workout clothes in various sizes—including petites and plus sizes—you want to pick out clothes that flatter your body shape. Clothes that are too tight can leave you feeling restricted. Clothing that is too baggy won't let you accentuate the parts of your body you should be proud of and can leave you overheated.

Some clothes have cool little hidden features, such as zipper pouches for keys, IDs, and phones. Some have built-in support that holds and lifts just where you want them to. Wearing clothes that you like will build your confidence and make working out that much more enjoyable.

Wear breathable fabrics. Certain fabrics are designed to breathe and wick away moisture as you sweat. They help keep the sweat off of you while you exercise, and they prevent chaffing or rashes. Cotton is a great breathable fabric but it will get wet quickly and stay wet. Look for fabrics made of spandex, lycra, polyester blends, wool, or polypropylene. You don't need to spend a fortune on workout clothes. Finding quality breathable active wear at most discount stores is easy these days.

Exercising in the dark? Wear reflective clothing. Companies have come to learn that it's safety first. Today you can find active wear with some kind of reflective element designed into it. Whether it's piping on the front, on the back, or along zipper lines, reflective clothing is in. Be safe and invest in a piece or two for those early-morning or evening walks or runs.

Wear a well-fitted sports bra. "Larger-breasted women can carry as much as five pounds per breast, making participating in high-impact activities like running difficult because of severe breast discomfort," says Elizabeth Goeke, executive vice president of Moving Comfort. Make sure you get measured and choose a supportive sports bra to ensure that you are getting the support you need.

MYplace **O** FOR FITNESS

Opt for color. No matter how much you love exercise, we all have days when we just can't get ourselves motivated or in the right frame of mind. Men and women alike, you don't have to always wear black anymore. For those days when you're feeling low or lacking in energy, why not invest in some vibrant-colored workout gear to help brighten up your workout? A colorful top with some slimming black capris, leggings, or shorts make for the perfect fun, upbeat and confident workout.

Let's face it, everyone looks slimmer in black, but as with women's fashion, men have more choices today too. Royal blue, red, neon green are great choices for that confident man. A good overall look for men is a mid-thigh-length relaxed pair of shorts over compression shorts, and a short-sleeved relaxed-fit shirt that adds a splash of color.

Opt for an updo. Girls, no matter how much you love wearing your hair down, at the end of a sweaty workout or run, you're not going to love this look quite so much. To keep your hair out of your face while working out, go for an updo, such as a high ponytail, braid or bun. To make sure it is completely out of the way (and to prevent it from getting sweaty), you could complete the look with a cotton hair band or a baseball hat made of wick-away fabric.

Guys, you too can grab that hat to help with sweat; or if your hair is long enough, try a top knot. Headbands and ponytail holders aren't just for women anymore. Accessorize. Adding some fun and useful accessories, such as a decorative water bottle, an exercise mat with a cool design, a sports watch, or a colorful gym towel and bag, is a great way to add some personality and fun to your overall look.

Makeup: yes or no? Some think that no makeup is the best way to go when working out, but others might feel they need to for a bit of extra confidence. The answer is a personal one, but exercise equals sweat, so if you do choose to wear makeup, opt for a light base of tinted moisturizer or mineral foundation. The last thing you want is heavy foundation running down your forehead and cheeks and being wiped all over your towel. Mineral makeup is especially good as it helps to reduce shine and provides the perfect coverage without blocking pores. Pair this with waterproof mascara and some tinted lip balm or subtle lip color for a natural look.

Spritz up with body spray. No time for a shower after class? A package of moist towelettes and some body spray will leave you feeling clean and fresh, and you won't have to worry about any unwanted smell as you run around town.

STAYING ACTIVE ON THE JOB

"Whatever you do, work at it with all your heart, as working for the Lord, not for men, since you know that you will receive an inheritance from the Lord as a reward"
—Colossians 3:23-24

Whether you work in the home, work from home, or work outside of the home, work is a necessary part of life. It can provide both joy and satisfaction. Unfortunately, it also brings schedules, deadlines, long hours, and many other responsibilities and stresses that can cause us to quickly spiral into a sedentary lifestyle.

A study in the Journal of Occupational and Environmental Medicine showed that workers who are moderately active get along better with their co-workers and take fewer sick days than their inactive counterparts. Highly fit employees perform more work than their colleagues—with little effort.[1]

The following are some tips to keep you active at work—even just 10 minutes at a time can make a huge difference in your overall wellness:

- Schedule physical activity just like you do important meetings.
- Park your car farther away from your office building.
- Take the stairs instead of the elevator.
- Use the bathroom on the next floor up or across the building.
- Deliver messages in person when possible.
- Take 10- to 15-minute walking breaks during your day, or schedule walking meetings.
- Stand up and do some stretching while you're talking on the phone.
- Buy some handheld weights or elastic exercise bands to use in your office.
- Go for a walk during your lunch hour.

MYplace O FOR FITNESS

- Start a walking group or exercise class at work.

- Make time for physical activity when you travel—walk in the airport between flights.

- Talk to your company about purchasing a few pieces of exercise equipment or implementing a wellness program. (Do your research about the benefits before making your request.)

REDUCE STRESS

You may not be able to eliminate the stress of your job, but you can learn to handle it in more positive ways. Stress often begins before you arrive at work: running late, taking care of personal responsibilities, and fighting traffic. Here are some tips to help you reduce stress and respond more positively to the stress you may experience on the job:

- Get organized; do most of your preparation the night before.

- Be sure to get enough sleep. Most people need seven to nine hours of sleep every night. Discover how much sleep you need and try to get it every night.

- Try to arrange your schedule so that you can avoid driving in heavy traffic.

- Leave your home early enough so that you're not rushed.

- Take time to relax before you leave for work or while you're in the car: breathe deeply, relax your muscles, pray, or listen to relaxing music or an inspirational message.

- At work, take 10 to 15 minutes once or twice a day to relax and organize the rest of your day.

- Prioritize your daily and weekly activities.

- Learn to recognize things that are less important or not important at all, and don't waste your time and energy on them.

- Schedule time for your own needs.

- Focus on one thing at a time.

- Learn to say no or "I need help."

- Personalize your workspace with pictures and special messages.

- Avoid cigarette smoke and limit caffeine intake.

- Look for ways to share responsibilities with your friends, co-workers and family. Think of specific things people can do to help you reduce your stress.

- Take time each week to discuss issues, plans, schedules and responsibilities with your family, friends and co-workers. Make this a time for teamwork and positive problem solving.

- Get away from work and take time for yourself and loved ones.

A SOOTHING BEDTIME ROUTINE

- Establish a relaxing nightly ritual—for instance, take a warm bath or read an uplifting devotional before you turn out the light. What kind of routine helps you wind down at night?

- Unplug from your electronics before you go to bed. Charge them away from your bedroom so that you aren't tempted to pick them up.

ARE YOU GETTING ENOUGH Z'S?

If you fall asleep within five minutes of lying down, then you are likely sleep deprived. How can you change your routine to make sure you get at least seven hours of sleep every night?

MYplace O FOR FITNESS

THE IMPORTANCE OF REST

I've heard it a thousand times: "Life just seems to be going faster and faster." We are busy people with busy lives. We live in a fast-paced world with so many things to do and so many places to be. The word "relax" means "to become loose or less firm, to have a milder manner, to be less stiff." "Rest" means "peace, ease or refreshment."

Why does God tell us to rest? Because it doesn't come naturally to us. In Genesis 3, the fall of man started a war against the life God had planned for us. Our need to control our lives has left us weary, tired, and without peace and refreshment. It has left us stiff.

Scripture draws us to a place of rest when it says, "Be still and know that I am God" (Psalm 46:10); "He makes me lie down in green pastures, . . . he refreshes my soul" (Psalm 23:2-3, NIV); and the most famous one in Genesis 2: "and on the seventh day God rested."

Jesus often drew away from the crowds to be alone, to spend time with the Father, and to pray. He is our example of how to live life well.

Many of us know what it feels like to stay up all night. We stay up with a sick child or loved one. There's a new baby in the house. We have work deadlines. Or we just have a sleepless night from time to time. But too many sleepless nights or staying perpetually busy can wreak havoc on our bodies.

God desires us to rest mentally. God desires us to rest physically. God desires that we would come and let Him take the cares of our world and lift our burdens so that we can rest. He wants to be all that we need, if we'd just let Him.

Rest is important to your health.

- Lack of proper sleep and rest has been linked to many health risks, including obesity, heart disease, and stroke.

- It prevents injury. When you push too hard without a break, your muscles and joints can become at risk for overuse injury.

- Overtraining can affect sleep. Too much training can put your body into a stressed state, which increases hormones such as adrenaline, making it difficult to sleep. Check your resting heart rate. Has it increased? Chances are you need to rest.

- It maintains a strong immune system. Without rest, your immune system can't make all the repairs it needs to your muscles and joints. The result is injury.

- It recharges you mentally. Have you ever suffered from burnout? It robs your desire to work out, enjoy family and friends, play, and enjoy life. Mental fatigue can be as detrimental as physical fatigue.

- Getting enough sleep and rest can encourage weight loss. It takes your body out of that stressed "fight or flight" state and allows you to recover properly.

Ask your family members if they think you are too busy. I guarantee they will be honest with you. When was the last time you spent a quiet time with God? Find time now. Invest in your relationships. Play with your kids; don't just be their taxi driver. Eat meals together and ask each other what the best thing was about the day. Slow down. Set aside time to recharge and refresh. Your life depends on it.

MYplace O FOR FITNESS

CREATING A FAMILY FITNESS PLAN

The statistics are staggering: According to the U.S. Centers for Disease Control and Prevention, only 21.6 percent of 6- to 19-year-olds in the U.S. reach 60 or more minutes of moderate to vigorous physical activity at least 5 days a week. Yet students who are physically active tend to have better grades, school attendance, cognitive performance, and classroom behaviors. What parent doesn't want that for their children?

So while you are creating a personal plan for health and wellness, why not involve the whole family and lay a foundation of health for your children, offering them all the benefits of being physically fit and blessing them with a healthy mom and dad.

Creating a family fitness plan can be a fun activity to do as a family. The following is a guideline to help you with this:

1. Step 1—Create your team. Call a family meeting. Get everyone on board from the beginning. Have fun with it. Come up with a team name. Discuss your current activity levels and talk about the things that can or should change. Commit to supporting each other and making this a fun adventure for the whole family.

2. Step 2—Commit to becoming more active together every day. Make a list of fun ways to exercise together. Make a game of it and come up with contests for those days when you can't be together. Design a family wellness contract or commitment. Include some of these activities:

   — Walk the dog together.
   — Play games together, such as tag, catch, jump-rope, or one of my personal favorites—hopscotch. Ask what they like best.
   — Ride bikes, rollerblade, or skateboard together.
   — Visit local parks or family-friendly recreation centers.
   — Go hiking.

3. Step 3—Plan meals together. Research has shown that the following are some of the positive benefits for children in families who eat meals together:

   — Better academic performance
   — Higher self-esteem

MY JOURNEY

- Greater sense of resilience
- Better family relationships
- Lower risk of substance abuse
- Lower risk of teen pregnancy
- Lower risk of depression
- Lower likelihood of developing eating disorders
- Lower rates of obesity

An added benefit for the *whole* family is that it saves money, which helps the family budget.

4. Step 4—Make and keep your family goals. Kids love stickers. Create a family-goals calendar and track your progress. Get the kids involved by letting them place the stickers on the chart, or let them create the chart. Accountability is key to staying on track.

Have fun and get moving!

MYplace O FOR FITNESS

BETTER TOGETHER—WORKING OUT AS A COUPLE

When it comes to exercise, men and women often participate in it differently. Men tend to pump iron, while women choose group fitness classes because of the social aspect. But can men and women work out together? And are there benefits to doing so? The answer is simple: yes!

Some of the couples I admire most are the ones who make it a priority to spend time together as often as they can. They play together, travel together, and some even work together! So, when it comes to fitness, why not grab your partner's hand and ask him or her to join you for a workout? Turns out, research has shown that couples who sweat together really do stay together.

Healthy Competition

My husband and I often laugh about how competitive we are. Truth is, we are. Using this competitive spirit in the gym or outdoors can be a fun way to improve speed and energy, and take your workout to a new level. A long-standing concept in social psychology is that the mere presence of someone else affects your ability to do an activity. Want to do more burpees? Have your partner join you for a workout.

Guaranteed Quality Time

Work, kids, and commitments take time away from time together as a couple. Fitting in a workout together can guarantee you some much-needed quality time together as well as allow you to stay fit. It's a great way to reap tremendous benefits as a couple and multitask by making yourselves a priority in body and soul.

Better Sex

One of the funniest lines from a movie is "Exercise gives you endorphins. Endorphins make people happy! Happy people just don't kill their husbands." Elle Woods had a point. Exercise brings on the symptoms of physiological arousal—sweaty hands, a racing pulse, shortness of breath. Endorphins are released when you exercise, which is why scientists say you feel better/happier after you exercise. But the release of endorphins also has other side effects, such as ramping up your sex drive and boosting your self-confidence. Need I say more?

Accountability

A study in *Prevention* magazine found that 94 percent of couples stuck to their workout plan when they did it together. It allows you to share in each other's successes and you'll keep each other motivated and get fitter in the process.

A Shared Goal or New Experience

New experiences flood your brain with dopamine, a feel-good chemical—and when you experience those things with your partner, your brain links that positive feeling with him or her. Similarly, when you share the goal of getting healthy and prioritizing your fitness, it becomes easier to achieve your fitness goals. The experience of being on the same page brings you infinitely closer.

A Deeper Emotional Bond

When you work out as a couple, you tend to match each other's rhythm, such as when walking, running, or lifting weights. This creates nonverbal matching, or mimicry. Nonverbal mimicry helps people feel emotionally in tune with one another. Those who experience or engage in it tend to report greater feelings of having bonded with their partner.

Workout Ideas for Couples

- Hit the gym or weight room together.

- Get outdoors. Go hiking, biking, kayaking, paddle boarding, rock climbing, or skiing together.

- Do a circuit workout together. Use one of the circuit workouts from this book.

- Go for a run or walk together.

- Take up a sport together, such as tennis, racquet ball, pickle ball, volleyball.

- Try a new activity together, such as ballroom dancing. It's fun, challenging, and romantic.

MYplace ○ FOR FITNESS

○ Bring on the competition and swim a few laps together, play a little one-on-one basketball, or how about a round of golf?

○ Take a group fitness class together, such as HIIT, boot camp, or kickboxing.

○ Relax together. Book a couple's massage or take a walk on the beach.

○ Pray together. Couples that pray together really do stay together.

CHOOSING HOME GYM EQUIPMENT

Life is busy, which means that the great thing about home fitness equipment is that it gives you the flexibility to work out anytime, regardless of the weather and without leaving the comfort of your own home. But before you run out and buy equipment, consider these time-saving suggestions to make sure that you get the most bang for your buck and that your purchase is the very best one for you.

Make sure the equipment is comfortable for you—otherwise, you won't want to use it. This is the most important factor aside from price. Can you adjust it for your body and exercise in the most comfortable position for you, standing or sitting?

Look for low-impact equipment. This means that it shouldn't put strain on your weight-bearing joints. Elliptical trainers and stationary bikes are good examples of this type of equipment.

Shop wisely. The equipment should be able to support your weight. Some pieces of equipment, for example, are only built to handle up to 210 pounds. Look for the recommended maximum user weight on the machine.

Make sure the equipment is simple to operate and has a safety button for stopping.

Try it out and ask for a demonstration of all the features.

Consider the manufacturer's warranty. Most home exercise equipment carries some type of warranty against defects in workmanship, which can range from 90 days for parts and labor to a lifetime warranty.

Make sure you have the proper space for it. There's nothing worse than investing time, money, and effort to purchase something that doesn't fit in your house. Before making your purchase, measure your space and learn how much space the machine will need around it.

Check Craigslist or online community yard sales. You can find nearly new equipment for sale by individuals who are tired of using it for a clothes rack!

Make sure you purchase something you enjoy using. Choose one that makes you want to jump on it 30 minutes of every day. Make an appointment on your schedule to fit your workout in. If you choose something fun, this won't be hard to do. If you are unsure if you'll use it or be consistent, consider renting equipment before purchasing.

MACHINE/EQUIPMENT TO CONSIDER

ELLIPTICAL CROSS-TRAINER: Elliptical machines provide total body conditioning, toning, and improvement of cardiovascular performance, and they are easy on the joints. Personal trainers have dubbed them the "most efficient way to burn fat and calories." They are a full-body machine, meaning they work the upper body, lower body, and core, and can adjust to your current level of fitness as well as to your future improved level of fitness. In particular, consider an Agile Dynamic Motion Trainer, a type of elliptical that is specifically built to cause less impact strain while providing over 12 body motions and 20 levels of exercise intensity.

REBOUNDER: This is a mini-trampoline that is easy on the joints and gives a great workout. Some come with a stabilizing bar to hold onto to do more intense workouts or to help you get comfortable on it when you first start out.

TREADMILL: This is, by far, the most popular piece of exercise equipment. The treadmill is versatile in that it offers both low-impact and high-impact workouts. Look for ones that adjust incline and speed. You want to be able to work toward a goal with a machine that will move toward that goal with you.

EXERCISE BIKES: This is a great choice if money is a consideration. Stationary bikes are usually less expensive than other exercise equipment and provide a truly non-impact option. There are upright or recumbent bikes. Recumbent bikes offer lower-back support and a more focused lower-body workout. Make sure to choose a bike that has an adjustable seat. Your goal is to be comfortable while working out. Bikes are a gentler option for the knees and joints.

FUN FOR THE WHOLE FAMILY: Consider Nintendo Wii, Xbox, or a fun dance game such as Dance Dance Revolution. Make memories you'll treasure for years to come and get fit all at the same time.

GYM-BAG ESSENTIALS

You have to get in a workout and then maybe go to the office or run errands. Besides your workout clothes and shoes, pack your bag with these few essentials to get you through all of your day's activities and leave you feeling clean and fresh.

Pair of headphones/charger—Music is one of the best motivators. Make sure you have everything you need to play those tunes as you work out. Must-haves: an extra charger for your phone, iPod, or MP3 player, and a pair of headphones or ear jacks.

Heart-rate monitor—Tracking your heart rate is a great way to work out effectively, maximizing your effort to make sure you are hitting your goals and not under- or over-training. Chest-strap monitors are the most accurate; however, almost all fitness trackers nowadays have them too. Keep it in your bag and you'll never be without it.

Deodorant—This is one of the most important things for your bag. No need to say more.

2-in-1 soap/cleansing cloths—At the gym and have little time for a shower? Save time by using soaps that combine hair and body wash or that combine shampoo and conditioner. No time for a shower? No problem! Just pack some disposable cleansing cloths to leave you feeling not so sweaty and smelly. Dry shampoo is another quick way to spruce up your hair in a hurry.

Shower shoes—This is a gym must-have and a simple solution to athlete's foot or other fungal diseases that are caused by warm, moist environments, such as in showers and saunas. An inexpensive pair of rubber flip-flops will do the trick.

Towel—Consider a "cooling" towel for your workout. These towels are specially designed to keep you from overheating during your workout and last for hours. If you plan on showering at the gym, keep a towel in your bag to dry off with if your gym doesn't offer them.

Water bottle—BYOWB (bring your own water bottle) with you. This is a great way to eliminate exposure to bacteria that linger around water fountains and it will keep you hydrated. A lot of community spaces, such as town centers, now offer filtered-water filling stations for runners/exercisers.

MYplace **O** FOR FITNESS

Disinfecting wipes/hand sanitizer—While the gym is a great place to get your workout in, it can also harbor bacteria on equipment surfaces. Most gyms offer disinfecting wipes for use before using a machine. If not, simply bring your own.

On-the-go snacks—Pack a few goodies to help you refuel and recover after your workout. A protein bar, a small bag of nuts, and a piece of fruit can all be easily stashed away in your bag for an end-of-workout treat.

Small makeup bag (women)—Save the makeup for after your workout. Makeup can clog your pores as you exercise—and who wants mascara running down their face as they sweat through a tough workout? If you have to wear makeup, consider a waterproof mascara and a light moisturizing foundation. Keep them in your bag for your post-workout routine and add a nice lip color to take you through your day.

Hair accessories—Before the workout: Keep bangs and flyaways under control with headbands. Ponytail holders will keep the rest in check. After the workout: a brush or comb for styling. Or, ladies, grab a hair clip and clip it up for a quick and cute updo look.

Band-aids/blister aids—Having a few band-aids or blister aids on hand can be an invaluable tool for those unexpected and unwanted blisters that can come during a workout.

Note: If you find yourself early for an appointment or waiting for your child's soccer practice to finish up, grab your tennis shoes out of your gym bag and go for a walk! Take advantage of the time.

STAYING ACTIVE WHILE TRAVELING

Let's face it, everybody travels. Whether it's for business, a weekend getaway, or a family vacation, we all find ourselves in a new city, country, or environment. And with that change in surroundings, our very normal routine gets interrupted and thrown out the window. For most people, our lives are pretty predictable. We are creatures of habit. We get up at the same time, have meals at the same time, go to bed at the same time, exercise at the same time. So how do we keep our exercise on track in a new and unfamiliar place and overcome time zones that change our sleep patterns? We plan for it!

First, choose a hotel that will help motivate you to exercise by asking the following:

- Does it provide an exercise room and/or indoor pool?
- Are there safe walking paths nearby?
- Is there a mall nearby where you can walk?
- Are there local fitness facilities you can use?
- Do they rent athletic wear if you forget to pack something?
- Will they provide in-room exercise equipment? If so, what is the charge for this service?

Second, consider the following:

- Check the local weather conditions before you go so that you pack the right clothing.
- Be prepared for unexpected delays. Wear comfortable shoes or pack some tennis shoes in your carry-on bag. Walk the airport terminal while waiting for your flight—even 10 minutes of exercise will help.
- A growing number of airports now have fitness clubs either right in the terminal or in hotels attached to a terminal. Las Vegas McCarran Airport, for

MYplace O FOR FITNESS

example, has a standalone gym on-site for anyone who wants to squeeze in a workout. Day passes make this an affordable option for travelers.

o Carrying your own bags will not only save you some money but will also provide some unexpected strength training.

o Take along a jump rope, a resistance band, or lightweight dumbbells. These are easy to carry and don't add a lot of extra weight.

o Find workouts to do in your hotel room from your computer. Just about any type of workout, from yoga to HIIT, can be found on the internet today.

o Be flexible and anticipate changes. If the weather is bad, walk in a mall or go to an indoor fitness center.

Business Trips

Today's travel is a bit more challenging with flight delays at their highest it seems. Just this can throw off an already tight schedule and leave you scrambling to catch up. Planning time to exercise can be difficult, but it's not impossible. In addition to the list above, here are a few other tips that can help you stay on track with your fitness goals while still meeting appointments and work commitments:

o Getting up a little earlier is a great way to reset your internal clock and allow you to start your day off right. Use this time to get your workout in at the beginning of the day.

o Take the stairs instead of the elevator. This is a good rule to put in place whether home or traveling. One of my husband's co-workers would choose a restroom on another floor to use and then take the stairs to get there. It challenged my husband to do the same.

o Schedule activity into your day just as you would a meeting. Better yet, take the meeting outside and have a walking meeting. It will keep the meeting timely and you'll get the benefit of some exercise. You just might influence your colleagues or business associates to move as they see that physical activity is part of your lifestyle.

- Many business trips offer the chance to play golf. Take along your clubs or plan to rent a set and just bring your golf shoes.

- Like racquet sports? Challenge your business associates to a game of racquet ball, tennis or squash. It's a great way to build relationships and stay active.

Vacations

Traveling for pleasure is a great way to enjoy your health and fitness. Go for a hike in the mountains, walk along a secluded beach, bicycle through the countryside, or windsurf over the waves. Don't worry about following your typical routine; look for new and fun ways to be physically active.

- Local attractions, such as parks, zoos, nature trails, museums, and other activities, can provide opportunities to see the sights and get some exercise at the same time.

- Consider active vacations, such as a spa retreat specializing in fitness, a camping trip in a national park, or a cycling trip during autumn in New England or even abroad.

- Look for ways to be active with your traveling companions. Rent bicycles, skates or other recreational equipment. Many cities today offer bicycle rentals that you can pick up in one location, ride to your destination, and then return it there.

- Go on walking tours, especially if you're in big cities that offer a guide. It's often easier to stay active if you have the support of others.

Finally, when you travel, whether for business or pleasure, don't push yourself. If you're tired, then rest or sleep. Sometimes your body needs sleep more than exercise.

MYplace ○ FOR FITNESS

WHY AND HOW TO CHOOSE THE BEST PERSONAL TRAINER FOR YOU

A good personal trainer is worth their weight in gold. A bad one can be a nightmare. So why hire one? And how do you avoid the nightmare? Personal trainers are not only for the rich and famous, but they can be a big investment. So, before you sign on the dotted line, you want to make sure you're getting what you pay for.

Research shows that working with someone who can show you how to safely move through exercises and add the encouragement you need to keep going can improve your fitness and strength goals.

Here's what a good personal trainer will do for you:

○ Help you get started if you are new to exercise

○ Show you new ways to maximize your workout

○ Work with your special needs, if you have medical problems or physical limitations

○ Develop a program for time-challenged people.

○ Coach you in your weight-loss journey

Finding the Best Trainer

It's hard to beat word of mouth. If you have friends who have been satisfied with their personal trainer—and you have noticed significant results firsthand—ask for contact information. But remember: what works for one person may not work for someone else. They have to fit you.

A good personal trainer will usually offer a free workout or assessment. Use that opportunity to ask about the following:

Are they credentialed? Today, many trainers have a college degree in physical education, sports medicine, kinesiology, or some other fitness-related field. Every trainer should be certified by a reputable organization, such as the American Council on Exercise, the American College of Sports Medicine, the Cooper Institute, or the National Strength and Conditioning Association. CPR and First Aid certifications should also be current.

How experienced is the trainer and what kind of experience do they have? The quality of time spent practicing is more important than the number of hours a trainer may have logged. In other words: a trainer learns by working with clients and adjusting as they monitor what is and isn't working for their client. Ask about their kind of experience. Do they have any specialties? Do they focus in one area of expertise? Do they work with a wide variety of clients? You want a trainer who knows how to work with you.

What is their strategy for dealing with injuries or preventing injuries? Your trainer needs to know what your weaknesses are and be able to design a program to work around them. They will also know how to work toward injury prevention by strengthening any muscle imbalance, correcting form, and not pushing you beyond what you are able.

Does the trainer's schedule work well with yours? Choose someone who can work with you on the days and times you are available. If your trainer can't commit to a schedule that works for you, find one who can. Convenience is key.

Make sure the trainer has liability insurance. Look for a trainer who insures himself/herself against personal injury and property loss.

Ask up-front about the trainer's business policies. What does he/she charge per hour? As a general rule, the average cost in a metropolitan area is $50 an hour. While there is an expense, even one session might be what you need to develop a plan and increase your motivation. And, as I already mentioned, look for a trainer who insures themselves against personal injury and property loss. It shows wise business practice.

Do they offer packages? Typically, the fewer sessions you buy, the more each will cost. Ask about payment options. Ask whether full payment is expected up front, per session, or as installments over time. Make sure the package won't expire before you have a chance to use all of the sessions you paid for.

Do they have a refund policy? This is especially important at a gym. If your trainer is no longer employed there, for example, will you be able to get a refund for the sessions you paid for or will you be forced to continue with another trainer? If you are unhappy with your trainer, can you get your money back?

MYplace O FOR FITNESS

Do they offer multiple-client sessions? Group training is a great option and usually costs less per person. Exercising with a few friends is fun, encouraging, and might save you all money.

Do they perform fitness assessments, and how often? Fitness assessments, such as body fat, blood pressure, strength, flexibility, and endurance, will help measure your fitness level. Based on your results, your trainer can then design a safe exercise program for you. Assessments can be performed periodically to assess your improvement and to make adjustments for your new fitness level.

Do they have a cancellation policy? Many trainers will require 24-48 hours notice for you to cancel a session without having to pay for it.

Request client references. Call the trainer's customers to find out his or her strengths and weaknesses.

Reasons to Break Up with Your Trainer

Have you ever been to the hairdresser, walked away disappointed, and thought it might be time to find another stylist? Or maybe for you it's a car: You get excited about the purchase, but after a while the newness wears off and you're ready for another one. Sometimes there are reasons to end your relationship with your trainer.

Your trainer pushes you too hard. Your trainer should know how far to challenge you without leaving you injured, exhausted, or overly sore (soreness that lasts longer than a few days). If you are experiencing any of these and your trainer won't modify your workouts, it's time to consider a break-up. A trainer should challenge you but respect your limits and ensure your safety.

Your workout isn't personalized for you. Each of us is uniquely created. Our fitness levels and goals are too. Are you feeling like you are not receiving personalized routines or attention? Talk to your trainer and let them know how you feel. If they don't respond, it's time to consider a break-up.

You're not seeing results. Doing the same thing over and over again can result in your muscles getting used to the exercise, thereby losing its effectiveness. If, after adjustments or modifications to your routine, you still aren't seeing results, then you might consider finding a new trainer who might challenge you in new ways.

You're not happy with your trainer's attitude. If your trainer insults you, is consistently tardy, doesn't give you their full attention, or tries to sell you things, then find a new trainer—immediately!

You're ready to go it on your own. You have a great trainer who has taught you what you need to know to build your own fitness plan, but now you're ready to try it yourself. If you are comfortable, give a try. Your trainer will always be there for tune-ups or any advice you might need.

Bottom line: it's your body, your money, and your time. If you are experiencing any of the reasons we just talked about, it's time to have that talk. Be kind and respectful. Do what's right for you and your overall fitness goals. You deserve the best.

THE 10-MINUTE WORKOUT

1. Warm up for 2 minutes.
2. Pedal, run or swim all-out for 20 seconds.
3. Pedal, run or swim slowly and easily for 2 minutes.
4. Pedal, run or swim all-out for 20 seconds.
5. Pedal, run or swim slowly and easily for 2 minutes.
6. Pedal, run or swim all-out for 20 seconds.
7. Cool down for 3 minutes.

Do this 3 times a week, for a total of 30 minutes of weekly exercise.

MYplace O FOR FITNESS

THE 7-MINUTE WORKOUT

Do each exercise for 30 seconds, followed by a 10-second rest.

1. Jumping jacks
2. Wall sit
3. Push-ups
4. Abdominal crunches
5. Step-up onto a chair
6. Squats
7. Triceps dip on a chair
8. Plank
9. High knees, running in place
10. Alternating lunges
11. Push-ups with rotation
12. Side plank, each side

30-20-10 OR 10-20-30

1. Run (or bike or swim or row) lightly for 30 seconds.
2. Run moderately for 20 seconds.
3. Run at top speed for 10 seconds.

Repeat the sequence 5 times, then rest for 2 minutes and repeat the sequence 5 times again. This routine takes 12 minutes to complete. If you are already in good shape, add another round of 5 repeating intervals. The next day, try a lighter exercise before trying 10-20-30 again.

MY JOURNEY

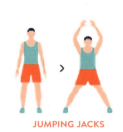 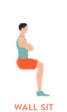 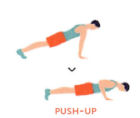

JUMPING JACKS   WALL SIT   PUSH-UP

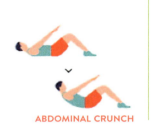 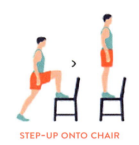 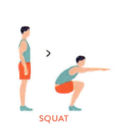

ABDOMINAL CRUNCH   STEP-UP ONTO CHAIR   SQUAT

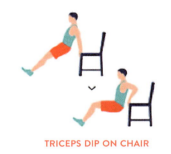 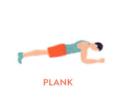 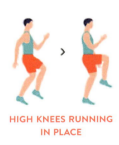

TRICEPS DIP ON CHAIR   PLANK   HIGH KNEES RUNNING IN PLACE

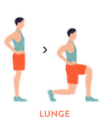 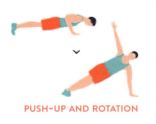 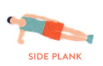

LUNGE   PUSH-UP AND ROTATION   SIDE PLANK

MYplace O FOR FITNESS

DATE:

sometimes the only difference between "try" & "triumph" is a little "UMPH"

I am **thankful** for . . . _____

_____

_____

_____

_____

my **live life fit** challenge is to . . . _____

_____

_____

_____

| # of minutes I was **active** today | my **energy** level today | O none | O | O average | O | O great |

today I feel . . . _____

_____

_____

_____

I **appreciate** this about my body . . . _____

_____

_____

_____

_____

My **inspiration** is . . . _____

_____

_____

_____

_____

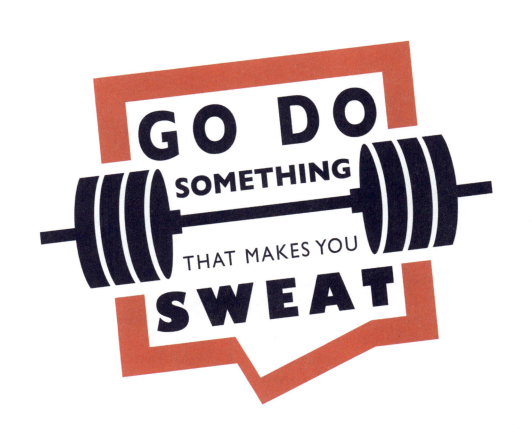

MYplace ○ FOR FITNESS

TURN OFF THE TUBE

A simple way to get off the couch and lose a few pounds at the same time is to turn off your TV. A recent study of the habits involving 5,000 National Weight Control Registry members (people who have lost an average of 73 pounds and have kept off at least 30 pounds for more than 6 years) revealed that most of them watch fewer than 10 hours of television a week.

AGE GROUP	TIME SPENT WATCHING TV/DVR AS OF 2016*
Ages 25-34	26 ½ hours per week
Ages 35-49	36 ½ hours per week
Those over 50	50+ hours per week

*According to Nielson ratings.

According to UC Davis Health, "Aerobic fitness (cardiovascular endurance) is the body's ability to deliver oxygen to your muscles, which allows them to do work or engage in activity. The lungs take in oxygen from the air we breathe where it gets perfused into the blood stream; the heart and blood vessels deliver it into the working muscles; and the skeletal muscles utilize that oxygen to execute muscular contractions and produce work." You might be asking, "Why should I care?" Because, according to the same article, "higher aerobic fitness levels are associated with numerous health benefits, e.g., longer lifespan, better quality of life, reduced risks for stroke, heart disease, diabetes and cancer, improved mood and self-esteem, and improved sleep patterns."[24]

> *Currently, however, public health data indicates that only 22-25% of Americans exercise regularly enough to achieve these positive health benefits.*

CAUSE FOR CELEBRATION

Here ar some ideas for celebrating your success:

- Make plans with friends to see a movie or go hiking.
- Buy yourself new workout clothes or shoes.
- Go on a weekend getaway.
- Treat yourself to a new piece of exercise equipment.
- Plan a dinner at your favorite restaurant.
- Get tickets to your favorite theater production or athletic event.
- Pamper yourself with a massage, manicure, or pedicure.
- Enroll in a class, such as ballroom dancing, yoga, art, painting, pottery.

"Wisdom is knowledge applied. Head knowledge is useless on the battlefield. Knowledge stamped on the heart makes one wise."

—Beth Moore

"Accountability separates the wishers in life from the action-takers that care enough about their future to account for their daily actions."

—John DiLemme

Whoever loves discipline loves knowledge, but he who hates correction is stupid

—Proverbs 12:1

I will choose Good over evil and will accept responsibility for my decisions

—Joshua 24:15

By wisdom a house is built, and through understanding it is established; through knowledge its rooms are filled with rare and beautiful treasures

—Proverbs 24:3-4

GLOSSARY OF FITNESS TERMS

What does it all mean? Here are some common terms to know about fitness:

A

Abduction: Movement of a body part away from the middle of the body. Standing with your feet together and lifting one leg to the side is an example of abduction.

Adenosine triphosphate (ATP): A high-energy molecule found in every cell. Its job is to store and supply the cell with needed energy.

Aerobic fitness: A measure of how well your blood transports oxygen around the body, and how well your muscles utilize the oxygen.

Aerobic exercise: An exercise where the oxygen demands of the muscles are provided by the circulation of oxygen in the blood.

Aerobic endurance: Ability to do prolonged exercise without fatigue.

Anaerobic exercise: An exercise for which the oxygen demands of the muscles are so high that the body can't replenish it quickly enough. As a result, the oxygen debt in the muscles forces the athlete to stop the exercise. Sprinting and weight training are examples of anaerobic exercise.

Athleisure: Refers to casual clothing—such as yoga pants, sweatpants, and hoodies—that is designed to be worn both for exercising and for doing (almost) everything else.

Atrophy: A decrease in size and functional ability of tissues or organs.

B

Beats per minute (bpm): The units of heart rate.

Basal metabolic rate (BMR): Estimates how many calories you would burn if you were to do nothing but rest for 24 hours. It represents the minimum amount of energy required to keep your body functioning, including your heart beating, lungs breathing, and normal body temperature.

Blood pressure: The pressure exerted against the inner blood vessel walls during heart contractions (systolic blood pressure) or during heart relaxation (diastolic blood pressure).

Body fat percentage: Simply the percentage of fat your body contains. If you are 150 pounds and 10 percent fat, it means that your body consists of 15 pounds fat and 135 pounds lean body mass (bone, muscle, organ tissue, blood, and everything else). A certain amount of fat is essential to bodily functions. Fat regulates body temperature, cushions and insulates organs and tissues, and is the main form of the body's energy storage.

Body Mass Index (BMI): An assessment of your weight relative to your height. The formula is: weight in kg / (height in meters x height in meters). The results of the BMI calculation are categorized as follows:

- Underweight: below 18.5

- Normal weight: 18.5-24.9

- Overweight: 25-29.9

- Obese: 30-39.9

- Morbidly obese: 40 and above

The BMI formula does not take into account your body composition (percent muscle vs. fat) and is therefore less accurate if you have a non-typical amount of muscle. This is because while a person with an above average amount of muscle is likely to be healthier because of it, the formula simply interprets the added muscle as fat and overestimates obesity. Conversely, with older persons and others with a below average amount of muscle, it underestimates obesity.

Body composition: Refers to the components of the body. It is usually divided into two components: the amount of fat mass (weight) and the amount of fat-free mass (muscle, bone, skin and organs) in the body.

MYplace ○ FOR FITNESS

C

Cardiorespiratory: Concerning the heart and respiratory system.

Cardiorespiratory endurance: The same as aerobic endurance.

Cardiovascular: Concerning the heart and blood vessels.

E

Endurance: The body's ability to exercise with minimal fatigue. Often used with other terms such as endurance training, muscular endurance, and cardio-respiratory endurance.

F

Fartlek training: Training in which the pace is varied from a fast sprint to a slow jog.

Frequency: How often you work out—how many days did you do cardio?Strength-training?

G

Glycogen: The form in which carbohydrates are stored in the body. Primary sites for storage are the muscles and the liver.

H

Heart rate: A measurement of the work done by the heart, commonly expressed as the number of beats per minute (bpm).

High-Intensity Interval Training (HIIT): A type of interval training where one performs a short burst of high-intensity (or max-intensity) exercise followed by a brief low-intensity activity, repeatedly. HIIT workouts usually last for a shorter duration due to the intensity. HIIT workouts provide improved athletic capacity and *condition* as well as improved *glucose metabolism*.[23]

I

Interval training: A training session that involves repeated bouts of exercise, separated by rest intervals. Depending on the length of exercise and rest periods, it may be anaerobic or aerobic training.

L

Lactic acid: Anaerobic exercise produces lactic acid in muscle tissue during exercise, where its buildup can cause cramping pains.

M

Maximal oxygen uptake (VO2max): The maximum capacity for oxygen consumption by the body during maximum exercise. Also known as aerobic power or maximal oxygen intake/consumption. VO2max is commonly used as a measure of aerobic fitness.

Maximum heart rate (MHR): The highest number of heartbeats per minute (bpm) when exercising maximally.

Metabolic equivalent (METs): Exercise experts measure activity in metabolic equivalents. One MET is defined as the energy it takes to sit quietly. For the average adult, this is about one calorie per every 2.2 pounds of body weight per hour; someone who weighs 160 pounds would burn approximately 70 calories an hour while sitting or sleeping.

O

Overtraining: Excessive training without adequate recovery.

Oxygen consumption: Defined as one's ability to extract oxygen from the atmosphere via the respiratory system and transport it in the blood to the working tissues (e.g., muscles) for energy production by the oxidation of carbohydrate and fat.

R

Repetitions (or Reps): The number of times a lift or effort is made continuously, one after another, and without any rest.

Resistance training: Training designed to increase the body's strength, power, and muscular endurance through resistance exercise.

Resting heart rate (RHR): The number of heartbeats in one minute (bpm) when a person is at complete rest. A person's resting heart rate decreases as they become more fit.

Resting metabolic rate (RMR): The body's metabolic rate (rate of energy use) early in the morning after an overnight fast and a full eight hours of sleep. This is different from Basal metabolic rate.

S

Sets: A group of repetitions. For example, 8 to 12 repetitions of bicep curls equals one set.

Strength training: See "Resistance training."

T

Target heart rate (THR) The target heart rate is your ideal heart rate, or pulse, during physical activity. Your target heart rate is within 50 to 85 percent of the maximum heart rate, which is the highest heart rate you should have during exercise.

V

VO2max: Oxygen consumption/uptake by the body. The highest rate at which you can uptake oxygen is termed the maximal oxygen consumption (VO2max). Research has shown VO2max to be one of the most important determinants of aerobic or endurance performance.

GLOSSARY

BIBLIOGRAPHY

BP's Fuel for Thought on WordPress.com. (n.d.). Retrieved from https://bps-fuelforthought.wordpress.com/page/44/

Activity Pyramid [Digital image]. (n.d.). Retrieved from http://www.wellspan.org/media/3648/activitypyramid-2009.pdf

Lifestyle Physical Activity [Digital image]. (n.d.). Retrieved from http://www.ccsoh.us/Downloads/Ch06%20Lifestyle%20Physical%20Activity.pdf

Water. (n.d.). Retrieved from https://visual.ly/community/infographic/health/water

Doheny, K. (n.d.). "The Truth About Fat." Retrieved from http://www.webmd.com/diet/features/the-truth-about-fat#4

"Keeping Belly Fat at Bay" (2006, January 31). Retrieved from http://duke-magazine.duke.edu/article/keeping-belly-fat-at-bay

Alizadeh, Z., Kordi, R., Rostami, M., Mansournia, M. A., Hosseinzadeh-Attar, S. M., & Faliah, J. (2013, August). "Comparison between the effects of contin-uous and intermittent aerobic exercise on weight loss and body fat percentage in overweight and obese women: a randomized controlled trial." Retrieved from https://www.ncbi.nlm.nih.gov/pubmed/24049613, https://www.ncbi.nlm.nih.gov/pubmed/8963358

"RPE Monitoring" (n.d.). Retrieved from https://www.acefitness.org/fitfacts/pdfs/fitfacts/itemid_2579

Fischer, D. V., & Bryant, J. (2008). "Effect of Certified Personal Trainer Ser-vices on Stage of Exercise Behavior and Exercise Mediators in Female College Students." Journal of American College Health,56(4), 369-376. doi:10.3200/jach.56.44.369-376

Mazzetti, S. A., Kraemer, W. J., Volek, J. S., Duncan, N. D., et al. (2000). "The influence of direct supervision of resistance training on strength per-formance." Medicine & Science in Sports & Exercise,32(6), 1175-1184. doi:10.1097/00005768-200006000-00023

Feldon, D. F., Peugh, J., Timmerman, B. E., Maher, M. A., et al. (2011). "Graduate Students' Teaching Experiences Improve Their Methodological Research Skills." Science,333(6045), 1037-1039. doi:10.1126/science.1204109

"Rev up your workout with interval training." (2015, March 24). Retrieved from http://www.mayoclinic.org/healthy-lifestyle/fitness/in-depth/interval-train-ing/art-20044588?pg=2

Gillen, J. B., Percival, M. E., Skelly, L. E., Martin, B. J., et al. (2014). "Three Minutes of All-Out Intermittent Exercise per Week Increases Skeletal Muscle Oxidative Capacity and Improves Cardiometabolic Health." PLoS ONE,9(11). doi:10.1371/journal.pone.0111489

"Really, Really Short Workouts." (n.d.). Retrieved from https://www.nytimes.com/well/guides/really-really-short-workouts?mcubz=1

Gojanovic, B., Shultz, R., Feihl, F., & Matheson, G. (2015). "Overspeed HIIT in Lower-Body Positive Pressure Treadmill Improves Running Per-formance." Medicine & Science in Sports & Exercise, 47(12), 2571-2578. doi:10.1249/mss.0000000000000707

Gibala, M. J. (2007). "High-intensity Interval Training." Current Sports Medi-cine Reports, 6(4), 211-213. doi:10.1097/01.csmr.0000306472.95337.e9

Reynolds, G. (2016, April 27). "1 Minute of All-Out Exercise May Have Ben-efits of 45 Minutes of Moderate Exertion." Retrieved from https://well.blogs.nytimes.com/2016/04/27/1-minute-of-all-out-exercise-may-equal-45-min-utes-of-moderate-exertion/

"Low-Volume Interval Training Improves Muscle Oxidative..." Medicine & Science in Sports & Exercise. (n.d.). Retrieved from http://journals.lww.com/acsm-msse/Fulltext/2011/10000/

Low_Volume_Interval_Training_Improves_ Muscle.5.aspx

Vincent, G., Lamon, S., Gant, N., Vincent, P. J., et al. (2015). "Changes in mitochondrial function and mitochondria-associated protein expression in response to 2-weeks of high intensity interval training." Frontiers in Physiology, 6. doi:10.3389/fphys.2015.00051

Gillen, J. B., Little, J. P., Punthakee, Z., Tarnopolsky, M. A., et al. (2012). "Acute high-intensity interval exercise reduces the postprandial glucose response and prevalence of hyperglycaemia in patients with type 2 diabetes." Diabetes, Obesity and Metabolism,14(6), 575-577. doi:10.1111/j.1463-1326.2012.01564.x

Massachusetts Institute of Technology (2013, October 15). "Ghrelin, a stress-induced hormone, primes the brain for PTSD." ScienceDaily. Retrieved from www.sciencedaily.com/releases/2013/10/131015191405.htm

Galland, M. L. (2011, January 13). "Leptin: How to Make This Fat-Burning Hormone Work for You." Retrieved from http://www.huffingtonpost.com/ leo-galland-md/leptin-how-to-make-this-fat-burning_b_806529.html

Genetic Science Learning Center. (2016, March 1) "Are Telomeres the Key to Aging and Cancer?" Retrieved from http://learn.genetics.utah.edu/content/basics/telomeres/

Van, K., Szlufcik, K., Nielens, H., Pelgrim, K., et al. (2010, November 01). "Training in the fasted state improves glucose tolerance during fat-rich diet." Retrieved from https://www.ncbi.nlm.nih.gov/pubmed/20837645

Aron, A., Norman, C. C., Aron, E. N., et al. (2000). "Couples' shared partici-pation in novel and arousing activities and experienced relationship quality." Jour-nal of Personality and Social Psychology, 78, 273-284.

Bond, C. F., & Titus, L. J. (1983). "Social facilitation: a meta-analysis of 241 studies." Psychological Bulletin, 94(2), 265-292.

Dutton, D. G., & Aron, A. P. (1974). "Some evidence for heightened sexual attraction under conditions of high anxiety." Journal of Personality and Social Psychology, 30, 510-517.

Fitzsimons, G. M., & Finkel, E. J. (2011). "Outsourcing self-regulation." Psy-chological Science, 22, 369-375.

Lewandowski, G. W., & Aron, A. P. (2004). "Distinguishing arousal from novelty and challenge in initial romantic attraction between strangers." Social Behavior and Personality: an international journal, 32, 361-372.

Skoyen, J. A., Blank, E., Corkery, S. A., & Butler, E. A. (2013). "The interplay of partner influence and individual values predicts daily fluctuations in eating and physical activity." Journal of Social and Personal Relationships, 30, 1000-1019.

Stel, M., & Vonk, R. (2010). "Mimicry in social interaction: benefits for mim-ickers, mimickees, and their interaction," British Journal of Psychology, 101(2), 311-323.

Zajonc, R. B. (1965). Social facilitation. Science, 149, 269-274.

Shisslak, C. M., Crago, M., McKnight, K. M., et al., "Potential Risk Factors Associated with Weight Control Behaviors in Elementary and Middle School Girls," Journal of Psychosomatic Research, March-April 1998, 44(3-4):301-13.

Bish, C. L., Blanck, H. M., Serdula, M. K., et al., "Diet and Physical Activity Behaviors Among Americans Trying to Lose Weight: 2000 Behavioral Risk Fac-tor Surveillance System," Obesity Research, March 2005, 13(3):596-607.

Serdula, M. K., Mokdad, A. H., Williamson, D. F., et al., "Prevalence of Attempting Weight Loss and Strategies for Controlling Weight," JAMA, 1999, 282:1353-1358.

Gimlin, Debra L., Body Work: Beauty and Self-Image in American Culture (Berkeley, CA: University of California Press, 2002).

Fairburn, C. G., and Cooper, Z., "Thinking Afresh About the Classification of Eating Disorders," International Journal of Eating Disorders, November 2007, 40(S3):S107-S110.

Marston, Stephanie, If Not Now, When? Reclaiming Ourselves at Midlife (New York: Grand Central Publishing, 2002).

ENDNOTES

KNOW YOUR FITNESS NUMBERS

[1] https://www.acefitness.org/fitfacts/pdfs/fitfacts/itemid_2579.pdf
[2] https://medlineplus.gov/ency/article/003399.htm
[3] http://dukemagazine.duke.edu/article/keeping-belly-fat-at-bay
[4] https://www.nhlbi.nih.gov/health/educational/lose_wt/risk.htm
[5] http://www.andjrnl.org/article/S0002-8223(05)00149-5/abstract

FITT TO BE FIT

[6] Gibala MJ, McGee SL. Metabolic adaptations to short-term high-intensity interval training: a little pain for a lot of gain? Exerc Sport Sci Rev. 2008;36(2):58–63.

Gibala MJ, Little JP. Just HIT it! A time-efficient exercise strategy to improve muscle insulin sensitivity. J Physiol. 2010;588(Pt 18):3341–3342.

Babraj JA, Vollaard NB, Keast C, Guppy FM, Cottrell G, Timmons JA. Extremely short duration high intensity interval training substantially improves insulin action in young healthy males. BMC Endocr Disord. 2009;9:3.

Whyte LJ, Gill JM, Cathcart AJ. Effect of 2 weeks of sprint interval training on health-related outcomes in sedentary overweight/obese men. Metabolism. 2010;59(10):1421–1428.

Nybo L, Sundstrup E, Jakobsen MD, et al. High-intensity training versus traditional exercise interventions for promoting health. Med Sci Sports Exerc. 2010;42(10):1951–1958.

Gillen JB, Little JP, Punthakee Z, Tarnopolsky MA, Riddell MC, Gibala MJ. Acute high-intensity interval exercise reduces the postprandial glucose response and prevalence of hyperglycaemia in patients with type 2 diabetes. Diabetes Obes Metab. 2012;14(6):575–577.

Guelfi KJ, Jones TW, Fournier PA. Intermittent high-intensity exercise does not increase the risk of early postexercise hypoglycemia in individuals with type 1 diabetes. Diabetes Care. 2005;28(2):416–418.

Maran A, Pavan P, Bonsembiante B, et al. Continuous glucose monitoring reveals delayed nocturnal hypoglycemia after intermittent high-intensity exercise in nontrained patients with type 1 diabetes. Diabetes Technol Ther. 2010;12(10):763–768.

Bassuk SS, Manson JE. Epidemiological evidence for the role of physical activity in reducing risk of type 2 diabetes and cardiovascular disease. J Appl Physiol. 2005;99(3):1193–1204.

Vella CA, Taylor K, Drummer D. High-intensity interval and moderate-intensity continuous training elicit similar enjoyment and adherence levels in overweight and obese adults.

Eur J Sport Sci. 2017 Oct; 17(9):1203-1211. Epub 2017 Aug 9.

Heinrich KM, Patel PM, O'Neal JL, Heinrich BS. High-intensity compared to moderate-intensity training for exercise initiation, enjoyment, adherence, and intentions: an intervention study. BMC Public Health. 2014 Aug 3; 14:789. Epub 2014 Aug 3.

Higgins S, Fedewa MV, Hathaway ED, Schmidt MD, Evans EM. Sprint interval and moderate-intensity cycling training differentially affect adiposity and aerobic capacity in overweight young-adult women. Appl Physiol Nutr Metab. 2016 Nov; 41(11):1177-1183. Epub 2016 Aug 10

Batacan RB Jr, Duncan MJ, Dalbo VJ, Tucker PS, Fenning AS. Effects of high-intensity interval training on cardiometabolic health: a systematic review and meta-analysis of intervention studies. Br J Sports Med. 2017 Mar; 51(6):494-503. Epub 2016 Oct 20.

ENDNOTES

STRENGTH TRAINING 101

[7] http://www.strongwomen.com/book/strong-women-stay-young/

[8] https://www.ncbi.nlm.nih.gov/pmc/articles/PMC3117172/

WATER: THE EVERYDAY GUZZLE

[9] http://www.webmd.com/fitness-exercise/features/water-for-exercise-fitness#1

[10] https://www.acefitness.org/fitfacts/pdfs/fitfacts/itemid_173.pdf

[11] https://www.ncbi.nlm.nih.gov/pubmed/14671205

[12] http://share.upmc.com/2014/09/importance-hydration-heart/

[13] https://www.ncbi.nlm.nih.gov/pubmed/21551998

[14] http://www.inaactamedica.org/archives/2013/24448328.pdf

[15] https://www.ncbi.nlm.nih.gov/pmc/articles/PMC2908954/

[16] https://www.ncbi.nlm.nih.gov/pubmed/21736786

[17] https://www.ncbi.nlm.nih.gov/pubmed/15953311

FIT YOUR FEET—10 TIPS FOR CHOOSING THE RIGHT ATHLETIC SHOE FOR YOU

[18] http://www.webmd.com/fitness-exercise/features/how-choose-athletic-shoes#1

[19] http://www.podiatrytoday.com/article/7784 Josh White, DPM

5 REASONS YOU AREN'T LOSING WEIGHT: PLATEAUS, STALLS AND ALL-OUT STANDSTILLS—HOW TO BREAK THROUGH

[20] https://www.acefitness.org/fitfacts/pdfs/fitfacts/itemid_2670.pdf

[21] https://jissn.biomedcentral.com/articles/10.1186/1550-2783-11-7

[22] https://www.scholars.northwestern.edu/en/publications/aerobic-exercise-improves-self-reported-sleep-and-quality-of-life

GLOSSARY OF FITNESS TERMS

[23] P. B. Laursen, D. G. Jenkins (2002), "The Scientific Basis for High-Intensity Interval Training," Sports Medicine (Review). 32 (1): 53–73. doi:10.2165/00007256-200232010-00003. PMID 11772161.

TURN OFF THE TUBE

[24] http://www.ucdmc.ucdavis.edu/sportsmedicine/resources/vo2description.html